Solving the
Depression
Puzzle

Solving the
Depression
Puzzle

*The ultimate **investigative** guide to uncovering the **complex causes** of depression, and how to overcome it using **holistic approaches***

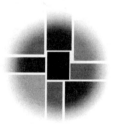

RITA ELKINS, M.H.

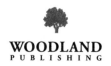

WOODLAND
PUBLISHING

Library of Congress Cataloging-in-Publication Data

Elkins, Rita.
  Solving the depression puzzle : the ultimate investigative guide to uncovering the complex causes of depression and how to overcome it using holistic approaches / Rita Elkins.
     p. cm.
Includes bibliographical references and index.
  ISBN 1-58054-095-3 (pbk. : alk. paper)
  1. Depression, Mental—Popular works. 2. Depression in women—Popular works. 3. Depression, Mental—Treatment—Popular works. 4. Holistic medicine. I. Title.
  RC537 .E35 2001
  616.85'27--dc21
                          00-012867

For ordering information, contact:
Woodland Publishing, P.O. Box 160, Pleasant Grove, Utah 84062
(800) 777-2665

Note: The information in this book is for educational purposes only and is not recommended as a means of diagnosing or treating an illness. All matters concerning physical and mental health should be supervised by a health practitioner knowledgeable in treating that particular condition. Neither the publisher nor author directly or indirectly dispenses medical advice, nor do they prescribe any remedies or assume any responsibility for those who choose to treat themselves.

First Edition

10 9 8 7 6 5 4 3 2 1

Printed in the United States of America

Please visit our website:
www.woodlandpublishing.com

CONTENTS

not to Eat: Food Choices to Prevent Sugar Blues • The Glycemic Index • A
Note on Artificial Sweeteners • Using Stevia as a Sugar Substitute •
Supplement Game Plan for Carbohydrate Metabolism Disorders

CHAPTER 8
Food Allergies and Mood Disorders

How Do You Define a Food Allergy? • Symptoms of Food Sensitivities •
Food Allergies Impact Behavior • Food Allergies Can Be Easily
Misdiagnosed • How Do You Become Food Intolerant? • A List of Foods
Commonly Associated with Allergic Reactions • Food Additives Recognized
as Safe by the FDA • What to Do if You Suspect a Food Allergy • Supplement
Game Plan for Treating Food Intolerance

CHAPTER 9
The Colon Connection to Depression

High-Protein Diets Create Colon Toxicity • What Constitutes
Constipation? • Colon Disease and Depression • Supplement Game Plan
for Treating Digestive Disorders

CHAPTER 10
The Female Face of Depression

Girls Tend to Become Depressed Early • Factors that Make Women More
Vulnerable to Depression • Stress and Cortisol • The Impact of Abuse on
Women • Hormonal Flux and Mood • Estrogen Dominance • Women,
Chocolate and Depression • Carbohydrate Cravings and Estrogen •
Vitamin B6 and L-Tryptophan for PMS Mood Slumps • The Link Between
Postpartum Depression and Vitamin B and Folic Acid Deficiencies •
Menopausal Mood Slumps • Supplement Game Plan for Hormonally
Driven Depression • The Profound Value of Exercise for Emotional
Problems Caused by Hormones

CHAPTER 11
The Light Link to Mood

Light and Biochemistry • The Melatonin Mood Link • How Does SAD

Make You Feel? · Food Cravings and Light · Children and SAD · Light Exposure and Vitamin D · Light Therapy is the Answer · Morning Light Exposure May Be Best · Other Interesting Facts about Light Therapy · Supplement Game Plan for SAD

All Sleep Isn't Necessarily Good Sleep · REM Sleep and Depressive Illness · Serotonin, Sleep and Depression · Hypersomnia: Too Much of a Good Thing? · A Kinder, Gentler Waking · Programmed Sleeplessness: A Surprising Treatment for Depression · Supplement Game Plan for Sleep Disorders · Dietary Guidelines for Improved Sleep · Supportive Therapies

Blame the Body · The Thyroid Connection to Depression · Dietary Guidelines for Low Thyroid Function · Supplement Game Plan for Dysfunctional Thyroid · Yeast Infections and Depression · Dietary Guidelines for Preventing and Treating Yeast Infections · Supplement Game Plan for Yeast Infections · Low Cholesterol Levels and Depression · Fibromyalgia, Pain and Mood · Supplement Game Plan for Fibromyalgia

Feeling Glum Can Literally Break Your Heart · Heart Rhythms, Blood Pressure and Depression · Depression Can Worsen Diabetes · Prolonged Depression Causes Bone Loss · Depression Can Increase the Risk of Stroke · Depression May Be a Marker for Alzheimer's Disease · Depression Can Weaken Your Immune System · A Final Word

Obesity as a Result of Emotional Stress · Obesity and Depression · Carbohydrate Binging: The Missing Piece · The Genetic Link to Eating

Acids: Fabulous Fats • Fish Oil and Psychiatric Disorders • DHA: A Special
Omega-3 Fatty Acid

C H A P T E R   2 2
"Exercise" the Demons of Depression 327

Exercise: No Better Antidepressant • You Can't Feel Sad and Exercise at the Same Time • Exercise Stimulates the Release of Mood-Boosting Brain Chemicals • Body Motion Oxygenates Brain Cells

C H A P T E R   2 3
Spiritual Healing 333

Dealing with Depression Requires Charity • Depression Numbs Our Spiritual Receptors • Patience and Empathy Are Vital • Faith Precedes the Miracle • Draw on the Powers of Heaven • The Very Real Therapeutic Power of Prayer

C H A P T E R   2 4
The Game Plan: An Overview 341

Become Proactive • The Antidepression Day-Plan • Beneficial Habits To Form and Maintain

Afterword 347

Bibliography 349

Index 357

Introduction

JUST A FEW years ago, I wrote a book titled *Depression and Natural Medicine*, which dealt with natural alternatives to conventional drug treatments in the fight against depression. In the short time since then, dramatic clinical data has emerged supporting the use of specific natural compounds to treat depression. Not only has St. John's wort created widespread interest as an herbal antidepressant, new substances such as SAMe, DLPA (DL-phenylalanine), and DHA (docosahexaenoic acid) are now emerging as credible treatments for mood disorders. In response to the large amount of new data on treating depression naturally, I decided to revisit the subject.

As I studied the latest depression research for this book, it became apparent that treating depression can be extremely difficult, whether you go to a physician or try to manage it on your own. Not only is our brain chemistry very delicate, it can also be affected by countless variables both inside and outside the body. Anything from constipation to prescription drugs and environmental toxins to hormones or food allergies can cause changes in mood. Because of the myriad of causes that can lead to mood disorders, if you suffer from depression, before you start any medication—natural or conventional—you may want to use what I call the "puzzle-solving approach" to depression.

The puzzle-solving approach is what it sounds like—a piecing together of factors that may be contributing to depression in order to find possible solutions. To use this approach, you will need to become a detective of sorts, using your problem-solving skills to analyze potential underlying causes for your depression. As you begin investigating these contributing factors, you may be surprised to find that the causes of depression are not as one-dimensional as you thought (or were told by your doctor). In fact, depression is often composed of numerous pieces, all contributing to the formation of a depressed state. This combination of factors can vary from person to person, but regardless of what is creating feelings of depression, this book will help you effectively evaluate your illness and determine hidden factors that may influence mood. It will also aid you in constructing an individualized solution for effectively and safely overcoming depression.

It is my belief that if you arm yourselves with the right facts about mood disorders, you will be able to not only uncover the causes of your depression, but also treat them more effectively. Many depressed individuals reach for their antidepressants without considering hidden physical conditions that may be causing them to feel low. And while pharmaceutical solutions for depression have met with some success, droves of depressed people are still looking for natural remedies to elevate mood. Natural solutions for depression are appealing because they are often less harsh and have fewer side effects. Moreover, natural medicine is known for its ability to treat the body as a whole rather than in parts.

When we treat the symptoms of only one part of the body, we are often ignoring reactions to the illness by other parts of the body, or we misread the causes of our symptoms altogether. Alternative practitioners are trained to see connections between problems throughout the body and to treat common causes, rather than merely treating symptoms specific to one part of the body. In fact, natural medicine has long believed that when one part of the body gets well, another seemingly unrelated part often also improves. This idea particularly applies to mood disorders and brain function.

Doctors are now discovering that many people who suffer from depression are responding to a variety of physical conditions that profoundly impact their brain chemistry. Everything from food to fungi can cause mood slumps. Becoming educated is the key to pinpointing the hidden biological culprits that may be causing your depression.

What you discover may surprise you. For example, a high-carbohydrate breakfast may be contributing to your afternoon mood slumps, or a chronic case of the blues may be the result of a thyroid malfunction. Depression may even be linked to prescription drugs taken to regulate blood pressure. You may even find that one factor for depression (like caffeine intake) won't affect your mood on its own, but when combined with other mood-altering factors (like sleep deprivation or hypoglycemia), it has devastating effects on mood.

In addition, low levels of chemicals like serotonin are not the only causes of depression. New evidence also recognizes malfunctioning electrical systems in the brain cell network as possible causes of depression. In fact, scientists are beginning to realize that the brain is similar in structure to a moldable piece of clay: its structure can actually change under certain circumstances. Moreover, if the brain fails to detoxify itself of old chemicals and metabolites, depression can result.

Whatever the contributing factors, you need to search them out. I was surprised to discover that both low and high estrogen levels can cause depression. Additionally, a deficiency of even one vitamin, mineral or amino acid can leave us feeling depressed, and blood sugar disorders like diabetes are also linked closely to mood.

What happens in the mind can affect the body and vice versa. In fact, being depressed can put you at higher risk for a heart attack, osteoporosis and even diabetes. This mind-body connection is often neglected in traditional circles of medicine, although the tide is changing.

Modern medicine typically limits itself to assessing symptoms and treating them with powerful chemical drugs. Until we see ourselves as a marvelous mix of the physical and the spiritual, however, we'll keep searching for that pharmaceutical magic bullet without success. The human body cannot thrive if its spiritual dimension is denied. Holistic health practitioners, no matter how primitive, knew this basic truth—so why don't most of us?

I must also add that twenty years ago a book like this would have had little chance of appearing on bookstore shelves. The notion that nutritive or herbal therapy held any value for the treatment of disease was considered a radical and irresponsible belief. Certainly no reputable professional would have jeopardized his or her credibility by advocating the validity of nonpharmaceutical therapies.

What we are seeing today is nothing short of a health revolution.

The consequences of stress, exposure to harmful toxins, our dietary habits, and our dependence on pharmaceutical agents to survive demand that we examine the value of natural medicine. The notion that mainstream medicine holds all of the answers is wavering. If the answer to our epidemic of depressive illness were solely the emergence of drug treatment, wouldn't we all be cured by now? The Prozac phenomenon, appearing in all of its "new and improved" versions, coupled with the widespread use of sleeping pills, anti-anxiety drugs, and tranquilizers has done too little to remedy the problem of depression.

In fact, one of the most common complaints people have about their doctors is that they don't take the time to address concerns, questions and possible causes of their depression. We need to ask more questions, explore more avenues, open more minds. To this end, I have divided the book into two main parts. In the first half of the book, I address key physical factors that may contribute to depression. In the second half of the book I examine the best natural compounds and therapies available for treating it. In addition, I have included specific treatment plans designed to target various physical disorders that may be responsible for your depression. These treatments can be taken in combination with a general treatment plan.

In this book you will find up-to-date discussions on the most effective natural remedies for depressive illness, dietary factors that may play a role in mood disorders, as well as the benefits of using magnets, acupuncture and other alternative therapies for mood boosting. New data in this book also reveals little-known links to depression, such as heart disease and cholesterol levels.

If you or someone you know suffers from depression, find out all you can about the disease and treatment options. Although most "alternative" or "natural" treatments are relatively unfamiliar to physicians, more and more of them are being used within the medical community and tested in research studies. The references, quotes and statistical data included in our discussion originated from reputable clinical studies, and the diet and nutritional breakthroughs presented in this book have their basis in scientific journals and medical records.

The goal of this book is to inform depression sufferers that not only do natural treatments exist, but that they also be very effective. All that is required of you is to become informed. Treatments work best when you understand your body and your illness. Applying the puzzle-solving approach to your depression will prepare you by making you more aware of how your body works and what factors influence how your body functions. Ideally, these approaches work best with the cooperation of your physician, but because you are ultimately responsible for your own health, you must take the initiative for gathering information that enables you to make educated choices.

Of course, it must be stressed that the information in this book is in no way a mandate for self-diagnosis or self-treatment. By all means, see your doctor if you feel depressed, but make sure your physician is well versed in both the conventional and alternative therapies available to you. Hopefully, this book will serve as a springboard for you and your doctor to plan the best treatment for your particular needs.

CHAPTER 1

Depression:
The Great Destroyer

*Man could not live if he were entirely impervious to sadness. Many sorrows can be
endured only by being embraced, and the pleasure taken in them naturally has a somewhat melancholy character. So, melancholy is morbid only when it occupies too much
place in life; but it is equally morbid for it to be wholly excluded from life.*

EMILE DURKHEIM

IRVING CAESAR ONCE announced that an optimist proclaims we live
in the best of all possible worlds, and a pessimist fears this is true.
Granted, life is difficult. Regardless of its obvious challenges, however, too many of us are suffering from serious depression. Why
does a pervading sense of melancholy haunt millions of people,
plaguing their lives with diminished purpose and performance
during the most prosperous time in our history? We have so much
to live for, and yet the good times have failed to chase away the goblins of depression. However, understanding the facts about what
depression is and who it strikes (and how) is an important first
step to recognizing and problem-solving your depression.

If you or someone you know feels depressed, you are certainly
not alone. Depression is the number one public health problem in
the United States, and it is on the rise. The National Institute of
Mental Health has estimated that over twenty million Americans
may be suffering from serious depression at any given time, and
another 5 percent feel down in the dumps. At least one person in

six experiences a serious depressive episode during their lifetime, and depression in young people is getting worse.

Depression is also costly—not only in terms of lost time, but also financially. Estimates place the economic price tag for depression at $43 billion a year (treatments, lost work days, etc.), and of course, the human toll is enormous. According to two articles published in the *New York Times*, an estimated 290 million working days are lost each year due to depression—a statistic that translates to $11.7 billion in lost productivity. To give you a better idea of the magnitude of this problem, the annual sale of antidepressants in the United States alone amounts to more than $3 billion. Globally speaking, over 330 million people are depressed, and most of them never get any treatment. Some estimates say that within the next two decades, depression will become second only to cardiovascular disease in worldwide scope.

The seriousness of this disease explains why being informed is so important. Any person who wants to take a puzzle-solving approach to their depression needs to first understand the myths surrounding the disease. For example, one prominent myth about depressed people is that they stay confined to their houses. Surprisingly, however, most people suffering from depressive illness don't take to their beds. On the contrary, 72 percent of depressed individuals remain in the workplace and try to tough it out with or without medication. And it is becoming more evident that the devastating effects of depression are not restricted to a certain class or type of people. Recently, Marie Osmond appeared on the popular *Oprah Show* to discuss the devastating effects of her postpartum depression. Other celebrities who have fought depression include Mike Wallace, Winston Churchill and Mark Twain.

Erich Fromm once said, "One cannot be deeply responsive to the world without being saddened very often." Feeling sad, however, and being depressed are not the same thing. This idea is another common depression myth that can be deadly. In fact, depression is a disease that can be fatal. Frequently, depression ends in suicide, despite the availability of antidepressant drugs. Sadly, tens of thousands of depressed people try to end their lives every year, and approximately 16,000 succeed in this country alone—and over

800,000 worldwide. According to the latest data from the Center for Disease Control's National Center for Health Statistics, suicide is the ninth leading cause of death in the U.S., after AIDS. In people aged 25 to 44, it is the fifth leading cause of death; and in those aged 15 to 24, it is the third leading cause of death, following accidents and homicides. In fact, in 1995, the number of suicides exceeded the number of homicides in this country.

Approximately 15 percent of patients who have depression for more than thirty days commit suicide. Many of these people have sought medical help within one month of their suicide. Every day, fifteen people between the ages of 15 and 24 kill themselves.

While the statistics are staggering, even more shocking is the fact that childhood depression is on the rise and adolescent suicide attempts are escalating. In the midst of unprecedented prosperity, why do great numbers of our young people feel compelled to waste their lives in hopelessness or even worse, to cut them short?

Modern Medical Practitioners and Depression

WHERE ARE THE DOCTORS?

One of the most alarming aspects of depression is that doctors frequently fail to recognize and treat it effectively. Depression often reveals itself in the form of headaches, back pain, bowel disorders, chronic fatigue, insomnia, chest pains and other seemingly unrelated physical symptoms. A recent report by the National Depressive and Manic Depressive Association found that 55 percent of depressed individuals are neither diagnosed nor treated by their family doctors. And if depression is suspected, an antidepressant drug is commonly prescribed. While these drugs can help, they come with significant side effects, and the quickness with which conventional doctors prescribe these drugs is troubling. In his book *Toxic Psychiatry,* Dr. Peter Breggin states:

> [M]inor tranquilizers, barbiturates, opiates, alcohol and perhaps antidepressants' effects are short lived, with little or no evidence for

sustained relief, and the hazards are considerable, including addiction, withdrawal reactions, rebound anxiety, mental dysfunction and lethality. Few psychiatrists would keep a pitcher of martinis at hand in the office to ease the anxiety of their patients; yet most are willing to reach into the drawer for a sample of 'alcohol in a pill,' the minor tranquilizers. Both . . . accomplish the same thing—a brief escape from intense feelings by suppressing or sedating normal brain function . . . should doctors endorse this dangerous and self-defeating avenue as a form of medical treatment?

We live in a society that is quick to medicate itself without looking into the whys and wherefores of disease. Certainly, modern medicine saves countless lives by using technology and pharmaceuticals—very few people would argue that point. However, in our vigorous attempt to treat depression with the latest drugs, many doctors overlook the profound impact of therapies that instead utilize diet, natural compounds, light and exercise.

By ignoring or minimizing these options, physicians often fail to get to the root of the problem in their depressed patients. In many cases, that solution is found in seemingly unrelated body systems that are out of balance. Additionally, our spiritual and emotional health are often ignored in traditional medicine. That is beginning to change, however.

In the remainder of the chapter, I discuss some groups particularly vulnerable to depression. Understanding why these individuals are more likely to suffer from mood disorders may help you solve the puzzle of your own depression.

Baby Boomers and Depression

A statistic in the *Archives of General Psychiatry* tells us that the rate of clinical depression has been steadily increasing in each succeeding generation born since 1915. We have to ask, what effects two world wars have had on our societies? On top of the wars we have been exposed to in this century, some have speculated that baby boomers are experiencing a delayed reaction to the social climate of the fifties and sixties, which saw unprecedented rates of divorce and the acceptance of a new kind of morality.

Prosperity also comes with an emotional price tag. The fact that baby boomers grew up in a never-before-seen time of economic boom may have led to rampant materialism. The restlessness and lack of fulfillment that have emerged in the last few decades only proves the old adage that money can't buy happiness. The psychological consequences of "keeping up with the Joneses," like the resulting envy and competition, may be more serious than we imagined. Pressure is high and so is the risk of disappointment. Peggy Lee, who sang the blues like no other, put it well when she asked, "Is that all there is?"

Consider also that post-World War II lifestyles have increasingly demanded more from successive generations and offered less in terms of good nutrition, emotional support and spiritual grounding. It's also true that pollution, poor eating habits, eating disorders and the time spent in closed, badly lit and badly ventilated environments have increased since the 1940s.

Eating disorders alone afflict enormous numbers of middle-aged and young women. Moreover, eating overly processed and highly sugared foods has become the rule rather than the exception. Much of the food we consume today (and for that matter, over the last several decades) has been chemically altered and unnaturally preserved. In addition, we're now eating nonfood substitutes as if they were the real thing. Aspartame, saccharin, fake fats, artificial textures and colors are casually ingested with no real thought given to their long-term effects. Most of us assume that if the FDA says it's okay, then it is.

Teenage Risk on the Rise

As mentioned earlier, adolescent depression has skyrocketed over the last few decades, and suicide is the third leading cause of death in teenagers. Our teenagers are in serious emotional jeopardy. Among college students, suicide is the second leading cause of death. According to the American Psychiatric Association, it is estimated that over 5,000 teenagers commit suicide every year. Facts that could shed some light on these staggering statistics came from a study on teenage suicides. The study found that most of these teens had deplorable eating habits and, in many ways, were malnourished. The typical teenage diet consists of caffeine, white sugar, alcohol, large amounts of fat, empty calories and junk foods. We know that without certain nutrients, the brain cannot function normally. It's not difficult to see that eating habits like these wreak havoc on the human body and mind, especially during periods of high stress (which characterize most of adolescence). In fact, stress actually leaches nutrients such as the B vitamins out of the body.

In addition, eating disorders and starvation diets are common behaviors among our young women. The need to stay thin often propels these girls into extreme diets that can deplete necessary nutrients and cause emotional stress. This vicious cycle can wear down resistance and alter mood. The lower our nutrient levels are, the less we can cope with stress. And the more stress we experience, the lower our nutrient levels become. Adding malnutrition to other adolescent stressors (social acceptance, dysfunctional families, grades, financial pressures, etc.) makes for a dangerous mix.

The Elderly Epidemic of Depressive Illness

And our young are not the only ones at risk. Getting old has become synonymous with sadness in our culture today. Unfortunately, depression is one of the most challenging problems we see among the elderly. Dr. Barry D. Lebowitz, chief of the Mental Disorders of the Aging Research Branch of the National Institute of Mental Health, cites figures that indicate thirty-three million Americans age sixty-five and older suffer from depression. He points out that depression is a primary concern in nursing homes and other care facilities, including medical units of hospitals.

In his work, Dr. Lebowitz emphasizes that depression should not be viewed as an inevitable consequence of getting older. He points out that depression is not normal and should not be thought of as an acceptable reaction to physical illness, misfortune or aging. In fact, depression can actually cause premature death in the elderly. Lebowitz notes that depression commonly exists side by side with other diseases—stroke, Parkinson's disease, heart disease, and fractures.

Suicide is also considered a major risk factor for the elderly, especially if their depression goes untreated. Dr. Lebowitz tells us that from 1980 to 1992, the suicide rate among persons age sixty-five and over increased by 9 percent. He writes, "Most striking was a 35-percent rise in rates of suicide for men and women age 80 to 84. The suicide rate among elderly, white, 'oldest old' males (those 85 and older) is six times the rate of the general population. All but a handful of older people who commit suicide are suffering from depression."

Naturally, social isolation and loneliness play a role in depression for older individuals; however, the roles of malnutrition and overmedication are rarely addressed. Frequently, older individuals lack key nutrients that influence brain chemistry—couple that with the potent drugs most older people take every day, and you have a recipe for mood disorders.

Typical American Eating Habits and Mood

We also now know that the consequences of the typical American diet on physical health are staggering to say the least. If 75 percent of the deaths in this country are due to lifestyle-related diseases, what percent of mental illness is directly influenced by the same factors? No one really knows. The relationship between lifestyle and mood disorders is only beginning to be uncovered, but a link between the two definitely exists.

There is no question that a nutrient deficiency can profoundly affect mood and mental outlook. In other words, if you become deficient in certain nutrients, your ability to cope can be impaired. In fact, your vision of reality may be significantly distorted. Moreover, there is new evidence that what we eat impacts our mood. The profound effect of our food choices on our mental and emotional state is addressed more fully later in the book.

American Immigrants and Mental Illness

Another factor of depression is explored in Roy Palmer's article "Is Americanization Depressing?" published in *The Daily Apple*. In the article, Palmer explores the idea that the American way of life can depress newcomers to the United States. He cites a University of California at Berkley study showing that Mexican immigrants who come to the United States become more vulnerable to depression. The study involved 3,000 individuals of Mexican descent living in this country. The study suggests that the longer an immigrant lives in the United States, the higher his or her overall risk for mental illness. In fact, rates for depression were four times higher for Mexican-Americans than for native Mexicans. In his article, Mr. Palmer stresses the idea that the traditional Mexican family structure provides a buffer against the hardships of immigration, poverty and poor education.

Naturally, what this suggests is that the breakdown of the family may be a primary contributor to mental conditions like depression—and not just for immigrants. I believe this study illustrates the idea that human beings need strong familial ties to survive in this world. Family support and love can provide emotional armor against life's upheavals. Even in America we are not guaranteed happiness—only the right to pursue it.

Social Issues and Emotional Health

Krishnamurti once said, "It is no measure of health to be well adjusted to a profoundly sick society." He may be right, but staying grounded in a culture that suffers from multiple ills is what this book is all about. Without a doubt, our society is suffering in many ways. For example, family stability is becoming a thing of the past. Like it or not, many of us live in households that are less than ideal.

Clearly, single parenting is one of the most difficult challenges anyone could face, and unfortunately, many parents and children are not given the support systems they need.

In addition, monetary pressures, behavioral problems, conflicts with spouses or ex-spouses, dissatisfaction with our appearance or status, and ordinary fatigue can make our lives seem hard to bear. Under these circumstances, it's no wonder we're inclined to feel blue. When the going gets so tough that the mind and spirit break down, depression can work its way into our psyches, and before we know it, we lose ourselves.

However, even in the most difficult of circumstances, if we are armed with the right tools we can overcome depression. The fact that depression rates are lower among married people—particularly married men—and the fact that people in long-term intimate relationships are depressed less often, tells us that companionship is a great deterrent to depression. In fact, depression is highest among divorced people and those who live alone—two groups that makes up a large part of nearly every neighborhood.

If you find yourself (or someone you love) in one of these groups, seek help and make the necessary changes to give yourself or your loved one the best possible advantage against depression. Those things that cannot be changed must be managed; however, in order to manage successfully, we must become as healthy as we can possibly be—both physically and spiritually.

Spiritual Famine

I must emphasize that in the course of doing research on health-related subjects over the last ten years, I firmly believe that the healing of any disease, including depression, must be based on respect for ourselves as miraculous entities—entities whose spirits and bodies are intrinsically interwoven. Disease is a disruption of a delicate biological balance, and healing must come from prompting forces that help both our spiritual and physical selves to get well from within as well as from without.

Within the last thirty years, the link between spirituality and health (and the pursuit of happiness) has largely been neglected. Because many of us are sensitive to religious and political issues, making reference to deity in public forums has all but disappeared. And although I support the separation of church and state, what has really happened in our society is the separation of people from God. I believe that a lack of spiritual focus in our society contributes to our feelings of dissatisfaction and frustration.

For generations, holistic medical practitioners taught that people cannot be healthy (or happy for that matter) unless all parts of their beings are nourished. In many ways, our souls have taken a beating. They have been abused or—even worse—ignored.

Certainly many of us have been disappointed with our lives at some point. Some of us are confused or troubled by issues of sexuality, intimacy, moral values, marital discord and the search for meaning in our lives. New studies tell us that when our spirits are hurt, our brains respond with actual physiological changes that determine how we feel. Recent scientific evidence suggests that we cannot separate our minds from the actual structure or mechanism of our brains. They have a mutual effect on each other.

And our society as a whole has lost its spiritual compass and replaced it with cynicism and materialism. The results have been catastrophic. The disintegration of love, both familial and marital, has resulted in the deterioration of our relationship with deity. So many of us feel as though we've become estranged from our God, especially when we feel depressed. When we let that happen, we become unfamiliar with the language of the spirit and deprive ourselves of a marvelous healing dimension.

Unfortunately, if you want spiritual support today, you have to seek it out. It is not as readily available as it used to be. Television, for example, a medium with the power to regularly fill our homes with uplifting and supportive programs, usually only serves to worsen our outlook on humanity. Movies and television shows rarely lift us, and sadly, the movie house has taken the place of the church house for many of us. More often than not, films are full of violence, perversion, discord and gratuitous sex. Our society literally thrives on dark amusement. Sunday night at the movies offers us a visual menu complete with murder, incest and infidelity.

As corny as it may sound, all of us need to get a good daily dose of something uplifting and wholesome. We are starving our spirits, and the price we are paying is a terrific one. I am grateful for celebrities like Oprah Winfrey who are not ashamed to openly acknowledge and build our spirituality. On many a gloomy afternoon when my heart was filled with dark thoughts, her show lifted me out of the depths. She uses the airways to work miracles in the lives of people who hurt. What do you think would happen if more producers took her lead? What if the evening news had to use half of its broadcast time building up the human spirit by inspiring human interest stories?

Depression among Russian people illustrates how lives without spiritual purpose and support can dwindle into self-destructive behaviors—suicide in Russia has dramatically increased since 1991, and so has its rate of alcohol abuse. When you take the human spirit and numb its desire to learn, produce, succeed and thrive, the results are nothing less than devastating. Yes, we know that depression is caused by a myriad of factors, but I will venture to say that it can also be a sign that our spirits have been neglected too long. Perpetual sadness can signal a longing for something that is not of this world. (For more on the spiritual side of depression and natural healing, refer to Chapter 23.)

New Perspectives on Depression

This book hinges on what diet, alternative treatments and spiritual recognition can offer victims of depression. Most of us believe that drug therapy is the only effective method for treating mood disorders. However, something as simple as changing what and when you eat may be pivotal in treating your depression. The role of sugar, caffeine, cholesterol, vitamins, amino acids, herbs and various other physical factors should not be underestimated. These factors can adversely affect mood and influence behavior, but most of us rarely consider these hidden, everyday catalysts when choosing how to fight our melancholia.

Moreover, depression can also be the by-product of a number of abnormal conditions. Yeast infections, viruses, a faulty thyroid gland and exposure to toxic chemicals can lead to depression in certain individuals.

Ironically, nineteenth-century doctors viewed depression as the result of chemical imbalances, an idea thrown out by Freud and Jung, who categorized depression as a psychological disease created by an overactive conscience. Today scientific data supports the notion that biochemistry and genetic predisposition can cause depression. In other words, for certain individuals, certain experiences can trigger changes in brain chemistry that result in extreme sadness. The availability of antidepressant drugs reiterates the real connection between chemistry and mood. However, the premise of this book is that other valuable natural treatments for depression also exist, and they are much safer and often more effective than drugs. Becoming aware of what's out there and how these treatments work is the key.

Has the medical profession overlooked possible causal factors in their ardor to find a quick chemical cure for this malady? Have the roles of hormones, carbohydrates, excessive dieting, light deprivation or the psychogenic effects of hundreds of widely prescribed drugs been sufficiently investigated? In our zeal to cure ourselves, are we failing to get to the root of the problem? This book will help you problem-solve depression by exploring both common and lesser-known factors that may be contributing to *your* low moods, as well as guide you to a individualized plan to treat your depression.

CHAPTER 2

Are You Depressed?

There is no despair so absolute as that which comes with the first moments of our first great sorrow, when we have not yet known what it is to have suffered and be healed, to have despaired and have recovered hope.

GEORGE ELIOT

DEPRESSION IS NO respecter of persons. It can strike anyone at any given time and is the most common, most misdiagnosed illness in America. Keep in mind that depression often recurs. In fact, those of us who have been depressed once stand better than a 50 percent chance that we'll become depressed again.

I strongly believe that I have been seriously depressed without realizing it. I can remember weeks when I would hide in my house, alternating between gloomy and not so gloomy, assuming that certain flaws in my personality were responsible for my social withdrawal. Being depressed can sound pretty ominous, and many of us think we have to feel suicidal in order to be considered clinically depressed, but that is a common fallacy.

Additionally, we frequently mistake depression for all sorts of ailments—a phenomenon that is discussed in more detail throughout this book. In fact, many Americans suffer through depression without knowing it or without seeking treatment. However, if you experience sudden mood changes that create dramatic swings in your feelings or if you struggle with persistent or periodic changes in mood, you may be suffering from depression.

If you're down in the dumps more than you are up enjoying life, you're probably suffering from some form of depressive illness.

Everyone feels blue at one time or another, and occasional low moods can make it difficult to distinguish a true melancholia from a simple emotional slump. However, if sad feelings are intense or prolonged, if they appear for no good reason, or if you've forgotten how to be happy, it's time to take action. Taking action means carefully investigating your physical, emotional and mental condition. By seriously examining our moods and habits, we will be able to piece together solutions to our problems with more accuracy. Taking a puzzle-solving approach to depression allows you to examine your physical and emotional problems in more detail and gives you solutions customized specifically for you.

True depression is a disorder, not a normal part of everyday living. It strikes people of all nationalities, backgrounds and ages, and various life events can precipitate a period of depression. In a vast number of cases, however, depression develops for no apparent reason. For this reason, I decided to start this chapter by examining the basics of depression, namely, the kinds of mood disorders and their general symptoms. Let's begin our problem-solving by acquainting ourselves with depression in all of its varieties.

Dissecting Depression

The following are typical categorizations of depression:

Atypical Depression. In this depressive illness, a person seems to be able to experience pleasure if placed in the right circumstance but sinks into a depressed mood when he or she returns to their normal settings. Chronic fatigue and lack of motivation can fill the times between fun or amusing events. Moodiness is common along with oversleeping and overeating.

Bipolar I. This illness is characterized by dramatic mood swings ranging from severe lows to extreme highs (mania). A person who is experiencing mania may have excessive energy, and he or she may feel restless and unable to relax. In manic phase, the person can develop delusions of grandeur, impaired judgment and bizarre social behavior.

Bipolar II. In this state, the manias are milder (hypomania) and the lows can vary in intensity. A person experiencing hypomania may become extremely talkative and social; their thinking may be unusually sharp with periods of enhanced creativity. This temporary state of elevated mood will eventually give way to a low period.

Cyclothymia. This form of bipolar illness is characterized by sudden mood changes. A person suffering from cyclothymia may feel up one day and down the next. The moods are unpredictable and seem to cycle regularly. Hypomanias followed by low periods can also occur in this type of depression.

Dysthymia. This is the technical name for chronic mild to moderate depression. A person with dysthymia will usually function from day to day but does so without any pleasure or sense of purpose or worth.

PMS (Premenstrual Syndrome). Depression is related to hormonal changes and can cause irritability, nervousness, low energy, body aches and bloating. Typically, this type of depression occurs about one week prior to a woman's menstrual period.

SAD (Seasonal Affective Disorder). This illness is caused by a person's physical and emotional reaction to light and usually affects vulnerable people during the winter months. Low energy, fatigue and overeating may appear when the days begin to get shorter and there is less sunlight. People who suffer from SAD may produce an excess of melatonin—the hormone related to the body's sleep cycle and biological clock.

Unipolar Depression. This form of depression is characterized by alternating periods of depression and normal life. During unipolar depressive episodes, the person may feel mentally foggy, fatigued or unable to function. A person may experience only one or two episodes of this type of depression, or they may have multiple episodes spread throughout the course of their lifetime.

The Hidden Faces of Depression

It is estimated that approximately one third of all people with depression don't know they have it, and the majority of those that suspect they do fail to seek out help. Why does depression often go unrecognized? Possible reasons include the following:

1. True ignorance. You may consider your symptoms as normal.
2. Shame, guilt or fear may prevent you from seeing your doctor or confiding in a family member or friend.
3. You may assume treatment costs will be too expensive.
4. You may feel helpless or lack the initiative to take action, or you may assume that there is nothing out there that can help you.
5. You may assume you have another disorder, such as chronic fatigue or fibromyalgia.

How Does Depression Make You Feel?

Depression impacts our thoughts, feelings, behavior, appearance and physical health. It affects every aspect of our lives whether at home, in the workplace, at school or in social situations. Depressive illnesses can last for months or even years. If you are truly depressed, you can't shake yourself out of it. Self-discipline, self-talk, or mental exercises like "counting your blessings" can't conquer true depression. Depression is not a behavioral problem that stems from laziness or lack of focus. It is a legitimate disorder and should be treated as such. The social stigmas attached to depression have been steadily diminishing because of better education and the growing number of people who suffer from the disease. Like any disorder, recognizing that you have it is the first step to getting well. Moreover, chemical reactions in the tiny world of your cells may be the real reason you fight depression. The first step to recognition is learning the signs of depression.

Symptoms of Depression

Look over the following list, and if you suffer from five or more of these symptoms and if they persist for more than two weeks, you need to see your doctor or health care professional for treatment. Keep in mind that each person is different and that the severity of depression can vary. The following illustrate the range of symptoms that could indicate some form of depression:

- difficulty making simple decisions, concentrating or remembering facts
- drug/alcohol abuse (can mask depression or anxiety)
- eating disturbances that include a loss or increase in appetite
- excessive crying
- experiencing phobic behavior, such as a fear of being alone or anxiety attacks
- fatigue and malaise or a loss of ambition
- feelings of hopelessness and overwhelming pessimism
- feelings of worthlessness, helplessness or guilt
- hallucinations or delusions
- hypochondria (one may actually feel symptoms)
- loss of interest or pleasure in ordinary activities, including sex
- panic attacks
- persistent physical symptoms that do not respond to treatment, such as headaches, digestive disorders and chronic pain
- persistent sadness, anxiety or "empty" moods
- restlessness or irritability
- sleep disturbances that include insomnia, oversleeping or waking up too early
- thoughts of suicide and death, or any attempts at suicide
- weight loss or gain

Perceptions of a Depressed Mind

Regardless of which depressive symptoms you may have, self-hatred is often a driving force in your depression. It's difficult to concentrate when you feel low, and even simple decisions can seem overwhelming. Feelings of frustration, hopelessness and lethargy are common to depression. If you're a woman, you have the added challenge of hormonal factors that can further aggravate and intensify mood swings. Elayne Boosler says that when women get depressed, they either eat or go shopping. Men, on the other hand, invade other countries. While there may be both humor and truth in her assessment, women who are seriously depressed don't even feel like spending money.

Typically, depressed individuals feel dismal for several weeks. Pleasurable experiences like eating or romance seem empty and unsatisfying. Depression can leave you feeling like you're operating in slow motion. It fills its victims with self-doubt and makes them feel perpetually pessimistic about their futures. Depression drains energy and fills the mind with thoughts of self-destruction.

THOUGHTS GENERATED BY A DEPRESSED MIND

The mind of a depressed individual spawns thoughts and feelings that are not conducive with self-improvement or productivity. Such thoughts may include:

- Even when I'm with people, I feel terribly lonely.
- Every task, even something as simple as getting dressed, seems so hard.
- I don't matter and everyone would be happier if I was gone.
- I feel so tired all the time.
- I have no friends and I don't really want any; I don't like people.
- I'm a burden to my friends and family.
- I'm always tired and mornings are the worst time of the day.
- I need to run away, but there's nowhere to go.
- I wish I could escape myself.
- I wish I could just sleep time away.

Depression in the Workplace

Symptoms of depression in the workplace may be recognized as a decrease in productivity, an unwillingness to cooperate, a rise in safety problems, an increase in accidents, a variety of unexplained aches and pains, alcohol or drug abuse, missing school or work on a regular basis, and a persistent lack of energy.

- Life is a hopeless trip to nowhere.
- No one understands how I feel.
- Nothing is left that makes life worth living.
- Nothing matters.
- The world is a horrible place to have to live.
- Why doesn't anything seem fun or interesting anymore?

If you've experienced these feelings for an extended period of time, you've probably been depressed and may have even contemplated suicide. But there is hope. There are things that you can do. In fact, if you experience periodic mood swings, you may be able to effectively control your down times through dietary management and supplementation alone. The important thing is that you begin unraveling your depression and find solutions for it now.

It is also essential that you do not underestimate the power of diet and lifestyle in your treatment plan. From 1960 to 1989, the cost of health care in America escalated from $27 billion to $500 billion dollars and is still rising. Much of the money spent for health care went to treating diseases that are the by-product of bad eating habits and lack of exercise. While medical science has recognized heart disease and cancer as lifestyle-related disorders, mental disorders have been viewed from a different angle. It's time to change that perception. There is a growing body of evidence to support definitive links between mood and the body.

Distinguishing Emotional from Biological Triggers

When discussing the symptoms and causes of depression, it is also necessary to make an important distinction between depression caused by a traumatic event and depression without any obvious emotional trigger. The first type of depression, typically called reactive depression, results from an event such as the death of a loved one, divorce, loss of a job, or other life-altering events. People who have this form of depression will usually improve with time and may benefit from psychotherapy.

On the other hand, people with the second type of depression, called endogenous depression, cannot link their mood disorder to any specific event. They frequently fail to respond to psychotherapy and may find themselves unable to break out of their mental misery. If you fall into this category of depression, brain biochemistry may be the culprit, and it's up to you to take the necessary steps to help yourself.

Many people who suffer from a mild biochemical imbalance may only experience sporadic symptoms of depression. Since the symptoms are mild and do not occur often, these people may not worry about treatment; however, if they are thrown into a serious emotional crisis, they can be prone to severe depression. In these instances, their depression is the result of a combination of reactive and endogenous factors. Of course, if a person is dealing with true grief, they should not feel guilty. It takes time to heal.

THE RIGHT TO GRIEVE

Experts used to say that the grieving process following the loss of a loved one should be expected to last for at least one year before its symptoms could be interpreted as clinical depression. Today, if a grieving person goes for eight weeks without snapping out of it, antidepressant drugs are readily prescribed. Granted, sometimes these drugs are needed; however, the process of grieving is an important one and should not be artificially cut short unless symptoms become extreme.

We live in a society that not only denies aging and death, but also wants to shorten or side-step emotional pain. Granted, during the first year after a loss, your doctor may recommend taking an antidepressant drug such as Zoloft or Prozac. For some people, this course of treatment can help them get through those difficult months. However, long-term side effects or dependency should be taken seriously when considering drug therapy. Consider trying SAMe or St. John's wort in combination with ginkgo and B vitamins for a more natural mood boost. If their effects fail to provide you with the lift you need, then talk to your doctor about pharmaceutical preparations. Keep in mind, however, that grieving in and of itself is a process that is beneficial in the long run and needs to be experienced.

Depression and the Body

Whether your depression is reactive or not, it is important to realize the connection between physical ailments and mood disorders that are becoming increasingly apparent in medical research. In fact, it is easy to mistake depression for other ailments, like unexplained aches and pains or consistent digestive disturbances. Depression can masquerade as persistent headaches, backaches, muscle spasms, sleep disturbances, chronic fatigue, constipation or changes in weight.

As I mentioned earlier, most depressed people don't recognize that they are depressed. Consequently, they may go from doctor to doctor describing an endless list of physical symptoms that have no apparent cause. The more doctors they see, the more medication they'll probably take, while the true source of the problem may remain unsolved.

In some cases, specific symptoms may be treated and even relieved; however, the underlying cause can often escape both patient and doctor. For example, chronic fatigue syndrome may, in reality, be depression disguised as consistent feelings of exhaustion. Likewise, a serious loss in appetite, insomnia or a decrease in weight may be caused by depression but attributed to stress.

Depression can also cause a wide variety of vague complaints, including the following:

• blurred vision
• dry mouth
• excessive sweating
• gastrointestinal problems (indigestion, constipation and diarrhea)
• generalized itching
• headache and backache

It is now widely accepted that depression not only accounts for a vast number of visits to the doctor's office, but is also frequently misdiagnosed and ill-treated. Frederick K. Goodwin, director of the National Institute for Mental Health, says that doctors who don't specialize in psychiatry recognize depression in only 25 percent of cases. He also admits that most physicians are likely to prescribe anti-anxiety drugs or sleeping pills that can act as depressants themselves, only making matters worse.

Donald F. Klein, director of research at the New York State Psychiatric Institute and coauthor of the book *Understanding Depression*, warns that many psychiatrists are not current in their knowledge of depression treatment, "being too wedded to lengthy psychoanalysis, perhaps, or unskilled in fine-tuning medication."

MYSTERY ACHES AND PAINS

There is no doubt that the body can reveal the state of your psyche. An article published in *The Journal of Clinical Psychiatry* reported that 41 percent of patients with depression go to the doctor with complaints of generalized illness. Thirty-seven percent of depressed people complain of pain, and 12 percent complain of general tiredness and fatigue.

Unexplained pain can be a marker of depression. For some people, coping with an emotional crisis means channeling mental anxiety into physical ailments, a process referred to as "somatizing." Part of the reasoning behind this phenomenon is the fact that depression makes you turn inward. In so doing, you can become acutely aware of your body. This unnatural preoccupation with your physical state can exaggerate physical symptoms, making them appear much worse than they really are.

PHYSICAL TRAUMA AND DEPRESSION

Just as physical symptoms can be signs of depression, physical trauma can lead to mood disorders in the first place. The human body operates best when all of its systems are balanced and working together in harmony. Everything that happens to us can disrupt that delicate equilibrium. Anyone who has had surgery or suffered a significant illness or accident understands this concept all too well. If you have recently had an operation or have struggled with a chronic or acute disease and became depressed, the assumption is that your depression is just an emotional reaction to physical stress. However, the very real biochemical effects of surgery, trauma, illness and drug therapy on the brain are rarely explored. You may be depressed because of a physical phenomenon. A kind of post-traumatic stress syndrome can occur after events like these. These factors should be considered when you begin to problem-solve your depression.

Unfortunately, misdiagnosing depression is not limited to how doctors interpret physical symptoms. A failure to see the link between mood and the body is common, but depressive symptoms such as anxiety, impulsive behavior, emotional stress and panicky feelings can also be misread by your doctor. Although these feelings are not always symptoms of depression, underlying mood disorders may not be considered when your doctor makes a diagnosis.

Excessive Worry and Anxiety

Being constantly worried or overly anxious about every day things can be a symptom of depression. Typically, depression can spawn persistent negative thoughts and phobias that predispose you to all kinds of exaggerated fears and anxieties. If you find yourself repeatedly waking up in the middle of the night and working yourself into a frenzy, you may be reacting to a disruption in brain biochemistry that can cause depression. You may spend the whole night stewing about something as simple as getting your car registration in on time, or you may worry about the potential threat of an earthquake.

Along with other symptoms, when you're depressed you can feel on edge, high strung or prone to panic for no apparent reason. Depressed individuals may feel unusually afraid in seemingly harmless situations. For example, they may drive across town to do some shopping and suddenly feel terror-stricken because they're so far from home. If something like this happens to you, see your doctor. Although his initial recommendation will probably be to begin drug therapy for panic disorders, don't be afraid to talk to him about alternative therapies that do not involve drugs. And remember—your panic may actually be a symptom of a depressive disorder.

Impulsive Behavior and Exaggerated Reactions

Although less common, doing wild, impulsive things like spending a great deal of money on trivial items or drastically altering your appearance can also be signs of a mood disorder. Frequently, because making choices seems so difficult when you feel depressed, individuals with mood disorders are often inclined to make bad decisions, which only serve to lower self-esteem. Something like picking the wrong color of paint or ordering something from the shopping network that you don't really need may lead to a serious emotional low.

After battling depression for extended periods, a small irritation can seem like an enormous calamity. A family friend who fell prey to this faulty perception of reality committed suicide one Sunday morning after the towel rack in his bathroom fell off the wall. In his mind, this seemingly insignificant event toppled a whole mountain of emotional stressors and pushed him over the edge.

The Wakefield Questionnaire

Before problem-solving your depression, take the following test known as the Wakefield Questionnaire. It is used in places like the University of Wisconsin medical school and can help you assess your particular mental state. It can also help you evaluate symptoms of depression that you may have overlooked. I believe it is one of the better tests. Read each statements and then circle the number in front of the statement that best describes how you feel now or in the last few weeks.

A. I feel miserable and sad.
(0) No, not at all
(1) No, not much
(2) Yes, sometimes
(3) Yes, definitely

B. I find it easy to do the things I used to do.
(0) Yes, definitely
(1) Yes, sometimes
(2) No, not much
(3) No, not at all

C. I get a very frightened or panicky feeling for apparently no reason at all.
(0) No, not at all
(1) No, not much
(2) Yes, sometimes
(3) Yes, definitely

D. I have, or feel like having, weeping spells.
(0) No, not at all
(1) No, not much
(2) Yes, sometimes
(3) Yes, definitely

E. I still enjoy the things I used to.
(0) Yes, definitely
(1) Yes, sometimes
(2) No, not much
(3) No, not at all

F. I am restless and can't keep still.
(0) No, not at all
(1) No, not much
(2) Yes, sometimes
(3) Yes, definitely

G. I get to sleep easily without sleeping tablets.
(0) Yes, definitely
(1) Yes, sometimes
(2) No, not much
(3) No, not at all

H. I feel anxious when I get out of the house on my own.
(0) No, not at all
(1) No, not much
(2) Yes, sometimes
(3) Yes, definitely

I. I have lost interest in things.
(0) No, not at all
(1) No, not much
(2) Yes, sometimes
(3) Yes, definitely

J. I get tired for no reason.
(0) No, not at all
(1) No, not much
(2) Yes, sometimes
(3) Yes, definitely

K. I am more irritable than usual.
(0) No, not at all
(1) No, not much
(2) Yes, sometimes
(3) Yes, definitely

L. I wake early and then sleep badly for the rest of the night.
(0) No, not at all
(1) No, not much
(2) Yes, sometimes
(3) Yes, definitely

Add up the circled numbers for all twelve questions. If your score is fifteen or higher, you should make an appointment with your doctor. If your score was below fifteen but you still feel that you might be depressed, see your doctor anyway to discuss your symptoms. Recognizing and treating depression early can decrease the severity and length of depression. Make sure you tell your physician that you would like to explore natural treatments before you go on antidepressant drugs. Finding a doctor who is willing to explore natural avenues of treatment is discussed at the end of this chapter. The important thing is to seek treatment immediately. Depression not only is a risk to your health—it can cost you your life.

Depression's Worst-Case Scenario: Suicide

Every year, 30,000 suicide deaths occur in the United States, and the number one cause of suicide is untreated depression. Furthermore, the actual number of suicides is thought to be much higher than statistically represented since suicides are often misreported as accidental deaths. Make no mistake—if depression is not addressed, it can be fatal. The *Journal of the American Medical Association* tells us that 95 percent of all suicides occur when depression is at its worse. A depressed mind distorts reality. Depressed individuals may begin to think that suicide is the best answer for everyone involved. A suicidal person does not believe that anyone or anything can help them. They just want out.

Patricia Slagle, a medical doctor who battled depression herself and wrote the book *The Way Up From Down*, points out that 82 percent of depressed patients who killed themselves had seen their physician within one month of their deaths. Fifty-five percent of them died of an overdose of tranquilizing or sleep medication supplied by the doctor. A current report on depression from Johns Hopkins University stated that antidepressants are the fourth leading cause of drug overdose and the third leading cause of drug-related death. Dr. Slagle goes on to say that she believes doctors would be wise to suspect depression in anyone with sleeping problems or anxiety.

All of us need to be aware of the warning signs that could signal suicide. We need to know how to identify those who may be preparing to take such a final and tragic step. Education is the key to prevention.

SIGNS OF SUICIDE

The following list provides an overview of signs that could indicate suicidal thoughts and feelings:

• buying a gun
• drastic mood swings or personality changes
• family history of suicide or any previous suicide attempt
• frequent drug or alcohol use
• giving away personal possessions or putting affairs in order
• having several accidents resulting in injury or close calls with death
• neglecting personal hygiene, finances, pets, etc.
• overwhelming feelings of hopelessness
• preoccupation with death in art, music, books, etc.
• recent trauma
• referring to reuniting with people who are deceased
• self-destructive or risk-taking behavior
• social isolation that is usually self-imposed

• statements implying that everyone would be better off without that person around
• sudden calm or uplifted mood after period of depression
• talking or joking about suicide
• unusual visits to people
• verbal or written references to suicide
• weight changes
• withdrawal from everyday activities
• writing morbid letters, poems or notes with a final theme

What Can Be Done to Prevent Suicide?

If you suspect someone is in real trouble, calmly ask them if they are considering suicide. Be empathetic but stay objective and nonjudgmental. If the person affirms your suspicions, ask them if they have decided how and when they want to die. Suicide threats should always be taken seriously. It's vitally important to stay with the individual who is seriously contemplating suicide, especially if they already have a plan. Insist that they come home with you, or immediately take them to see a doctor or counselor. If you know someone who has been suicidal and has overcome the situation, contact them for an immediate talk with the depressed individual.

Don't try to lift the person's spirit by talking about how good they really have it or pointing out all they have to live for. This often results in a more depressed state. Reassure them that there is help, that many others have felt this way, and that suicide is not the answer. Reiterate the fact that these feelings are just temporary and that making such a final decision is certainly not a good idea. Repeat back to the person what they are sharing with you, and stress to them that you are there for them and that you care. Call a professional for them and accompany them to their appointment. Use a suicide hotline if you have to and keep in close contact.

For more information on suicide prevention contact:

SA\VE—Suicide Awareness\Voices of Education
P. O. Box 24507, Minneapolis, MN 55424-0507
Phone: (612) 946-7998
Internet Address: http://www.save.org
E-mail: save@winternet.com

Finding the Right Doctor

Of course, the best way to prevent suicide is to treat depression before it becomes serious. One of the first steps in treatment is seeing a doctor. Many depressed individuals will not see a doctor, however, because they do not want to take expensive medications. Sir William Osler said, "One of the first duties of the physician is to educate the masses not to take medicine." It's troubling that currently, medical school criteria is sadly deficient in nutritional education but keeps on top of all the latest pharmaceutical drugs. Consequently, most doctors will discourage you from trying supplements or herbs.

However, not all doctors are like this—there is a growing contingency of medical doctors who advocate nutritional medicine. You just have to find one. I know what you're thinking. If you feel depressed, you're not going to want to go shopping for the right doctor. *Do it anyway—it could change your life.* Check local medical societies that may list physicians who use nutritional medicine or orthomolecular psychiatry. The Huxley Institute for Biosocial Research in Boca Raton, Florida, may also be able to supply you with the names of doctors who specialize in nutritional medicine, or get online and do some research of your own. Call reputable chiropractors and health clinics for recommended physicians. It's vital that you find a nutritionally oriented physician who is willing to discuss the information contained in this book.

Before making an appointment, ask the receptionist if this particular doctor is willing to use supplements as part of treatment. It may take several calls and inquiries to find a reputable doctor who believes that nutritional therapies are sound, but it will be better in the long run. Also, when you first see your doctor, clearly explain that you would like to treat your depression without using drugs. Talk about alternative therapies that you believe would be benefit you most, and then ask him to help you implement whatever strategy you choose. Increasing numbers of medical doctors are becoming intrigued by alternative treatments. Believe it or not, there are several doctors who openly praise the advantages of natural treatments over pharmaceutical drugs for diseases like depression.

Put natural medicine to work for you. Weigh all your options and be willing to look at the very real impact of diet, exercise and supplementation. The American Holistic Medical Association is comprised of medical doctors and osteopaths who believe in treating more than just the symptoms of disease. Write to the address below for names of physicians in your area that are members of this organization.

American Holistic Medical Association
4101 Lake Boone Trail, Suite 201
Raleigh, North Carolina 27607
(919)787-5146

The American Association of Naturopathic Physicians (AANP) is another professional organization that lists licensed naturopathic physicians in your area:

The American Association of Naturopathic Physicians
P.O. Box 20386
Seattle, WA 98102
(206)323-7610

How Good Is Your Doctor?

If your doctor is the kind of physician who spends very little time with you, is quick to pull out the prescription pad, and scoffs at any natural remedy, it is time to find yourself another one. Learn

An Interesting Note on Depression and Doctors

Ironically, when it comes to depression, the old adage "physician heal thyself" is particularly appropriate. Recent studies suggest that medical doctors are peculiarly susceptible to depression due to high stress and job burnout. Both factors negatively impact the brain chemicals that control mood. Emotional exhaustion and withdrawal are not uncommon among doctors—a fact that reiterates the very real effects of prolonged periods of stress on brain chemistry and mood.

to look for certain traits when you go shopping for a doctor. Find one who is willing to utilize the best of both conventional and natural approaches. When you go in for your first visit, use the following guideline to determine if your doctor is right for you:

• Do you feel rushed, uncomfortable or tense in the presence of your doctor?
• Do you like and respect your doctor?
• Does your doctor ask questions about your lifestyle, for example, your medical history, eating and exercise habits, stress levels, relationships, and any drugs/supplements that you may be taking?
• Does your doctor listen closely and give you ample opportunity to express yourself?
• Does your doctor respond well to your questions, no matter how trivial they may seem?
• Does your doctor seem genuinely interested in what you have to say and is he considering at least some of your desires when deciding on treatment?

Most importantly, use your intuition. Don't continue treatment with any doctor you are unsure of. Find one that will fulfill your needs. And if you are still seeing your family physician with chronic problems, ask him or her if depression could be your problem and who to see for treatment. If your doctor is unreceptive or curt, don't go back.

Most physicians will assume that your depression is either psychological, biochemical, or a combination of the two. Whatever your doctor believes is making you feel depressed, nutrition is often ignored. You probably won't be asked if you have any particular food cravings, or if you use caffeine or take vitamin supplements. For this reason, it is imperative that you seek out an openminded physician who is willing to help you plan a treatment strategy based on your particular psychological and physical needs.

Take Action Now

Most importantly, if you believe you are depressed, take action. If you can't, for whatever reason, ask someone you trust to get the ball rolling on your behalf. Although you may feel helpless and hopeless now, you don't have to go on that way. Today, more than ever, depression can be successfully treated and frequently cured altogether. If you're ashamed of your depression and believe that a social stigma accompanies the illness, think again. Depression is not your fault. It's a disorder like any other and is never a sign of weakness or lack of character. Depression can snag the heartiest and the best. Instead of wasting time denying your depression, get help right away. Life is too precious. Don't cheat yourself.

The first step to curing depression is to accurately diagnose the condition. This book will help you do that. Each chapter goes through specific factors that can lead to depression, as well as solutions based on those factors. This investigative approach will help you discover possible factors that could be affecting your mood. Make sure your doctor is willing to work with you when you begin analyzing why you are depressed and how to best tackle your problem. Good doctors will gather all the pertinent data they can to determine what's going on. Good luck!

CHAPTER 3

Mood: A Biochemical Balancing Act

Life is one, big, long chemical reaction.
UNKNOWN

As I MENTIONED in the last chapter, one of the most dramatic discoveries I made while writing this book is the complex interrelationship between physical, emotional and mental factors. For instance, a high-stress job, bad marital and family relations, and constant worrying about finances can all contribute to this complex interaction with physical factors (like sugar intake, hormones, light, exercise, etc.) to create a dramatic impact on the mind. Research is proving that the physical often determines the emotional—biological events can affect our emotional reactions and attitudes. The reverse also holds true—our moods can affect our physical health and our body's ability to function. Moreover, serotonin, the brain chemical most responsible for our moods, isn't working the way it should for many people. The purpose of this book is to help you uncover those physical factors that may be influencing your depression, so you can treat your depression at its source, not just treat its symptoms. But solving the depression puzzle can take some time.

Most of us probably only think of our brain as the seat of the intellect, rarely appreciating the fact that brain functions monitor and regulate all of our conscious behaviors like walking or thinking, as well as involuntary actions like inhaling and exhaling. The focus of this chapter is on how brain cells affect our emotions and sensory perceptions, and how they are affected by other body systems. Let's begin by taking a crash course on how the brain responds to stimuli.

1. The brain receives information from nerve cells called neurons from every part of the body.
2. It evaluates the information and sends appropriate instructions via the neurons.
3. Neurons communicate with the cells around it through electrical signals.
4. When a nerve signal reaches the end of one cell, it passes over a gap to reach the other one and causes the release of chemicals called neurotransmitters.

Any malfunction along this route may cause depression. In addition, improper detoxification of brain cells can trigger abnormalities that create feelings of depression. We also know that the brain stem controls sleep, and abnormal sleeping patterns (like sleeping excessively) can be linked to depression.

To date, medical scientists have concentrated on manipulating brain chemicals like serotonin, dopamine and norepinephrine with drugs to treat mood disorders. While this method has met with some success, we are beginning to understand that treating depression effectively may ultimately rely on treating other areas of the body that affect the way brain chemicals are released. The answer to the depression may not be a simple prescription. In fact, solving our mood problems often involves a detailed analysis into possible factors that need to be pieced together in order to find a solution. Let's begin by investigating some reasons why brain chemistry is important, and how it can get out of balance or work incorrectly.

Is a Gene to Blame for Depression?

As mentioned earlier, depression runs in families, suggesting that a genetic component can alter the way brain chemicals work, thereby making certain people more vulnerable to low moods. In fact, anyone with a family history of depression has a greater risk of becoming depressed than the general population.

In the past, researchers thought a single gene caused this susceptibility. Today, new data suggests that a group of genes is probably to blame. Canadian scientists have confirmed that several genes are responsible for both schizophrenia and manic depressive illness. Their research tells us that the genetics of a family line may predispose an individual to mental disorders such as depressive disease. One theory suggests that certain gene mutations can affect brain chemistry, which can make someone much more likely to feel depressed than another individual, even under the same circumstances. More research is currently underway; however, the fact that depression runs in families must continue to be addressed if we are to determine possible causes of mood disorders.

Depression: Brain Chemistry Gone Awry

The link between biochemistry and mood was first truly accepted during the 1940s and prompted the release of numerous antipsychotic and antidepressant drugs. New pharmaceuticals designed to change mood by manipulating biochemistry are hitting the market every year, and scientific findings then and now have unraveled quite a few confusions about biochemical reactions in the body and the brain.

For instance, we now know that the brain requires certain chemicals to function normally, and when the levels of these chemicals are disrupted, depression can occur. This neurochemical connection is called the "monoamine theory of depression" and has motivated the creation of several kinds of antidepressant drugs currently prescribed to millions of depressed individuals.

In addition, not only are the kinds and amounts of certain brain chemicals we have important, the sensitivity of certain receptor cells to the presence of these chemicals is also critical. Why? After brain chemicals or neurotransmitters are released, they attach to receptor cells that are designed to link up with that specific chemical alone. Imagine the chemical as a key and the receptor cell as the lock. In order for the door to be opened, the two must fit. When a fit occurs, it produces a certain effect. For example, some neurotransmitters excite, while others inhibit and minimize, emotion. Some transmit impulses that produce positive feelings of well being and others cause the development of negative or depressed sensations. And so, while it's important to remember that the quantity of these chemicals is important, if the receptor cells are impaired in any way, the key may be there, but the lock is missing or useless. Without both the key and the lock, the desired effect on mood cannot be achieved.

To illustrate how brain chemistry affects mood, let's examine one of the more well-known neurotransmitters, the endorphin. Endorphins have the ability to relieve pain and produce feelings of euphoria or contentment. Recent research suggests that sustained exercise can actually produce endorphins and create feelings of well-being. This reaction is typically seen in sports such as long-distance running. As mentioned earlier, endorphins bind to specific receptor cells in the brain.

Several other neurotransmitters are also responsible for regulating brain activity and functions that include not only mood control, but also memory, appetite, sleep and other functions. In most people suffering from depression, levels of neurotransmitters located in the mood-controlling areas of the brain are abnormally low. Consequently, these signals or impulses are not transmitted fast enough to adequately sustain normal mood. Antidepressant drugs address this problem by increasing the amount of these specific brain chemicals, especially one particular chemical, serotonin, which is discussed in various sections and chapters of the book.

NEUROTRANSMITTERS AND OTHER BODY SYSTEMS

Brain chemicals not only regulate mood, but also influence the secretion of hormones such as estrogen, progesterone, cortisol and melatonin. These hormones can influence mood as well. The connections between brain chemicals, hormones and mood illustrate an idea central to our discussion. Malfunctions in physical and mental health often sustain themselves by reacting to each other. Interactions among systems can create a loop where illnesses of one area can affect another area, which reinforces illness in the first area. For example, hormones can alter brain chemistry causing us to feel down, and the brain can affect our hormonal output, causing our moods to dip. Each problem feeds on the other. Deciphering our mood changes and the reasons for them, then, can often seem like a "chicken and the egg" dilemma. And in fact, we may never know which problem came first.

What we do know is that the brain tells us when we feel hungry, tired and sad. Why these signals become exaggerated in some people remains a mystery. Genetic blueprints that determine brain structure may be at the core of the problem. Be assured, however, that even if depression runs in your family, supplementing your brain cells with the right compounds can help to counteract this tendency.

NEW FINDINGS ON DEPRESSION: FAULTY BRAIN CIRCUITRY

Although mainstream science still considers brain chemistry the main culprit for depression, new evidence points to faulty electrical impulse transmission between brain cells as another contributor. Thanks to sophisticated technology, we can study the brain in much more detail than ever before. Some experts believe that depression results when brain cells break down, causing nerve connections to become "lazy." As a result, information is not processed properly. When this happens, responses that we would normally muster to cope with certain situations are simply not there. This theory is based on the idea that human emotions are governed to some extent by the nerve circuitry of our brains. If brain cell "wiring" is deficient, we may experience negative feelings.

What makes our brain electrical systems go haywire? One culprit is stress. There is compelling evidence that emotional strain can actually alter our brain's circuitry, which can change brain chemistry as well, consequently altering our mood. For example, some experts believe that childhood sexual or physical abuse changes not only the hormonal makeup of the victim's brain, but its structure as well.

Likewise, a depressed mind can actually destroy brain connections, making impulse transmission sluggish. This phenomena may explain why electric shock treatments (ECT) can sometimes "wake up" the brain and stimulate sleepy neurons, resulting in improved mood. This treatment is discussed in more detail in Chapter 4. Think of this electrical scenario as your brain trying to sustain mood, ambition and pleasure on low voltage. Put in simple terms, it needs a better power source or it fails to do the job. A lack of power can result in negative thoughts about everyone and everything.

CAN SLEEPY BRAIN CELLS SELF-DESTRUCT?

Furthermore, scientists are now suggesting that if the brain is understimulated, brain cells can die. And, as we discussed in the previous section, the way nerve cells in the brain transmit their signals regulates brain cells' performance. Once again, if levels of certain brain chemicals in these connections are low, brain cells can struggle to survive or even die off. The idea that depression may result from lapses in the way brain cells talk to each other is gaining ground. If we know that someone is at risk for this "slow transmission," we may be able to prevent depressive illness.

Is Depression Really Just a Physical Condition?

So, when all is said and done, is depression just a manifestation of a physical problem? There are a growing number of experts who believe that depression is really just a reaction to something else going on in the body. However, the reverse of this cause-and-effect scenario works as well. For example, did you know that a mood slump turns down the energy levels of organs besides the brain? In fact, when we feel emotionally low, we inadvertently set into motion a series of biological events that make all of our other body systems less efficient. And when our other systems aren't functioning up to par, our brain is affected, and we become more depressed.

What I find particularly compelling about these new theories is that they all support the belief that we cannot treat ourselves in parts. We must view ourselves as the sum of all our parts—physical, emotional, intellectual and spiritual. Unfortunately, the very things we choose to do or not do every day may be perpetuating the vicious cycle of depression.

Don't despair. Simply being aware of these interactions in your body is a promising first step. Why? Because now you have a greater awareness of how your body is supposed to work and how it is currently functioning. You now have a foundation to build on, a place to start your search for clues to your own mood. In the process of improving your mental well-being, you will enhance your physical health as well.

You May Be Your Own Worst Enemy

Many of us treat ourselves abominably. We routinely eat candy, chips, cookies, soft drinks and other sugary snacks to boost our sagging energy levels and scoff at the idea of food allergies and the damaging effects of food abuse. We remain oblivious to the chemical additives found in our foods, and treat ourselves to drinks loaded with caffeine just to keep ourselves going. We routinely skip meals, use pills to sleep and wake up, and work under a great deal of stress. But if somewhere along the line, we get a chronic case of the blues, do we know enough to connect our melancholia to our lifestyle choices?

The following scenario illustrates how various factors—physical, emotional and mental—can create and perpetuate a veritable depression cycle:

- Your job is stressful, and you regularly
eat snack food on the run.

↓

- You soon become deficient in B vitamins, which
lowers serotonin levels in your brain.

↓

- This causes you to feel tired, fatigued and depressed.

↓

- Coffee and caffeinated drinks are a favorite way to battle
your fatigue; however, the caffeine interferes with
normal brain chemistry, eventually causing you to
feel more depressed and lethargic.

↓

- You also regularly eat sugary snacks to give you more
energy, which makes your glucose levels unstable, adversely
affects serotonin levels, and depletes B vitamins. Your
depression, mental fatigue and lethargy worsen.

↓

- You soon find yourself in a virtual hibernation, finding it difficult get up in the morning, go to work, or even leave the house.

↓

- This "hibernation" leads to sunshine deprivation, which
causes your serotonin levels to dip further.

↓

- Your financial situation has been tight for some time.
You constantly worry about it.

↓

- Prayer and church attendance have been a regular part of your
life. Now both of those activities have slipped drastically.

↓

- Your spouse has become frustrated with your behavior; the
resulting arguments only add to already high stress levels.

↓

- You retreat more into a "shell," dwelling on the frustrations of work and home.

↓

- Throughout all this, your diet continues to worsen, and you have stopped exercising. Further inactivity, weight gain and lowering of energy levels result.

↓

- Your neglect of physical activity and poor diet have made you chronically constipated.

↓

- Constipation can lead to estrogen build-up, which creates anxiety and sleep problems. To help induce better sleep, you take a sleeping aid.

↓

- The sleeping pills only intensify your feelings of depression; maybe you reach for a drink. The alcohol depletes B vitamins and lowers serotonin levels.

↓

- Now your depression has become serious. Added to that, you lose your job because of poor performance . . . and the cycle continues.

This scenario should give an idea of the many and varied factors that can contribute to depression and related conditions. Some repeat themselves. Some are more influential than others. The point is that a puzzle-solving approach can be the best tool for finding the relevant pieces to your particular puzzle. Only then can you see the big picture and find a solution.

If you've learned anything about this scenario, it should be that we must become acutely aware of how our lifestyle choices affect our biochemistry. If we want to be happy, we have to be smart about those choices. Most importantly, if we've gotten ourselves into a vicious cycle such as the one described, there is still hope. By changing the habits that promote mood disorders, we can live happier, healthier lives.

CHAPTER 4

Conventional vs. Holistic Treatments for Depression

I will follow that system of regimen which according to my ability and judgement, I consider for the benefit of my patients, and abstain from whatever is deleterious.
FROM THE HIPPOCRATIC OATH

AN ESSENTIAL ASPECT to treating mood naturally is developing a keen sensitivity toward our biochemical selves and learning how that biochemistry affects our behavior. There are several natural ways to change the biochemical makeup of your brain, and by taking the "puzzle-solving approach" to recovery, you can determine the most effective changes for you. However, before you consider using any of these treatments, consult your doctor. And, if you are currently on prescription medication for depression, don't discontinue or modify your dosage in any way without your doctor's supervision. Take this book with you when you see your physician and tell him you want to try natural therapies. Remember to be assertive about your decision to try to get well naturally.

One of the greatest benefits of using natural medicine is that it empowers you to take responsibility for your own treatment. If you are intimately involved in the process of getting well, you gain more control over how you get well. You can listen to your body's responses to treatment and adapt to it accordingly. In order to take charge of your treatment, you need to know how to change your brain's chemical profile with the right supplements. But first, let's consider the differences between natural and conventional medicine.

The Philosophy of Natural Medicine

Voltaire said, "The art of medicine consists in amusing the patient while nature cures the disease." While his view may be a bit extreme, the crux of his quote is true: given the right tools, it's amazing how the body can balance and cure itself. Granted, some diseases get the best of us; however, natural practitioners base their treatment of disease on the idea that nature provides us with just about everything we need to get well. Unlike conventional medicine, which works from the outside in, natural remedies prompt healing forces from the inside out—a view that has met considerable skepticism from the medical profession. Regardless, the tried and true principles of natural healing are nothing new. For centuries they have been based on the following:

- Doing no harm to the patient
- Identifying and treating the cause of disease, not just its symptoms
- Promoting the role of physician as teacher as well as healer
- The healing power of nature

The healing approaches of traditional medicine compared with natural medicine are striking in their opposition. As you compare the two healing philosophies, think about depression as a disease.

Conventional Drug Treatments for Depression

The most commonly used conventional treatments for depression are antidepressant medication, psychotherapy or a combination of both. Psychotherapy can be helpful in uncovering behaviors or perceptions that may be contributing to your depression.

A Comparison of Health Care Philosophies

STANDARD MEDICINE	VS.	NATURAL MEDICINE
Considers the body as separate units	vs.	Considers the body a whole unit
Body and mind are separate entities	vs.	Body and mind are linked
Treats the symptoms of the illness	vs.	Finds and treats the cause of the illness
Attempts to eradicate disease	vs.	Promotes health
Uses drugs and surgery	vs.	Addresses diet and lifestyle
Physicians cannot be emotionally involved	vs.	Caring is vital to healing
Physician has the last word	vs.	Doctor works with patients
Physician is in control	vs.	Patient is in charge
The focus is on the objective	vs.	The focus is on the subjective

And in cases of moderate or severe depression, the first line of treatment is medication. Currently, antidepressants make up over $7 billion of the prescription drug market worldwide, and over the next five years, that figure is expected to double. Antidepressant drugs are all designed to manipulate certain brain chemicals like serotonin, norepinephrine and dopamine in order to elevate mood.

The rest of this chapter will explore why conventional treatments are prescribed, how they are supposed to work, and when you should consider employing or discontinuing their use. Hopefully, by becoming more familiar with the methodology behind conventional treatments for mood disorders, you will be able to better understand alternative treatments, and you will be able to make better decisions about what treatments are best for you. Don't be afraid to do further research on any or all of the treatments mentioned before making a decision to begin or halt a particular treatment. Being informed is essential to problem-solving your depression.

Why Does the Brain Fail to Supply Us with Enough Mood-Sustaining Chemicals?

For many of us, our brains lack the ability to sustain the chemicals we need to feel good about life. Several scenarios can explain impaired brain biochemistry. Below are a few of them:

• A poor diet can lead to a lack of compounds called amines that are used to make brain chemicals.
• An inherited condition can lead to an increased need for the necessary chemicals needed to manufacture these amines.
• Brain receptor cells may be impaired so that the amine is not received and converted into the right chemicals.
• Recycling processes in the brain may be faulty, leading to an excess of MAOs (monoamine oxidases) that may destroy too much of the brain's amine supply—this problem can be hereditary.

A Crash Course in Antidepressant Drugs

If your doctor prescribes antidepressant medication for your depression, it will most likely come from one of the following three categories:

1. Tricyclics (example: imipramine)
2. Monoamine Oxidase Inhibitors (MAOIs) (example: phenelzine)
3. Selective Serotonin Re-uptake Inhibitors (SSRIs) (example: Prozac)

Each one of these drug families takes a different chemical approach to alter brain chemistry, and it generally takes between three to six months after drug therapy starts to see results. Dosages are altered to suit specific needs and minimize side effects, and they should be monitored at regular intervals. Ideally, your doctor should inform you about the most common side effects associated with your prescribed drug; however, many doctors fail to adequately go over what to expect when you take a drug. Your physician should also ask you if you are taking any other medications that could cause negative interactions or if you're pregnant or nursing.

TRICYCLIC AND TETRACYCLIC ANTIDEPRESSANTS

Tricyclic antidepressants increase the brain cells' exposure to serotonin, which is what SSRIs do as well; however, the way that tricyclics accomplish this end is different from the SSRI process. This family of drugs is commonly used to treat moderate to severe depression and includes:

- amitriptyline
- clomipramine
- doxepin
- maprotiline (Ludiomil)
- nortriptyline
- trimipramine

- amoxapine
- desipramine
- imipramine
- mirtazapine (Remeron)
- protriptyline

Newer tetracyclics include maprotiline and mirtazapine.

Keep in mind that tricyclic medications are also prescribed for headaches, fibromyalgia, unexplained pain, and irritable bowel syndrome. These drugs should not be taken if you have glaucoma, benign prostatic hyperplasia (enlarged prostate) or certain types of heart disease. Tricyclic antidepressants can also produce adverse reactions in the cardiovascular system, including rapid heartbeat, high blood pressure, palpitations, abnormal heart rhythms and in some cases, heart attack and stroke. Psychiatric reactions include hallucinations, confusion, anxiety, nightmares, insomnia and disorientation. Other side effects include numbness, tingling, loss of coordination, ringing in the ears and seizures. If the drug is abruptly discontinued, nausea, headache and malaise may occur.

MONOAMINE OXIDASE INHIBITORS (MAOIs)

This category of antidepressant drugs influences the same neurotransmitters (serotonin and norepinephrine) that tricyclics do, in addition to the brain chemical called dopamine. The three brain chemicals we know as serotonin, norepinephrine and dopamine are also called monoamines. After they have performed their chemical function, these monoamines are metabolized by a protein in the brain called monoamine oxidase. Antidepressant drugs that are MAO inhibitors work to block this function. In so doing, excess brain chemicals stick around for longer periods of time and actually accumulate in brain cells. The design of these drugs is based on the belief that low levels of these monoamines can cause depression.

The downside to MAO inhibitors is that they cause an amine called tyramine to build up. As a result, your blood pressure can rise. In fact, too much tyramine can cause a sudden jump in blood pressure that can even be fatal in some people. In addition, certain foods—aged cheese, wine, yogurt, yeast extract, liver, some beans, chocolate and caffeine—produce more tyramine in the brain, so you have to avoid them while taking MAO inhibitors.

In the 1960s, when this class of drugs hit the market, no one knew about the tyramine risk. Consequently, a number of deaths from brain hemorrhages occurred. This effect is called hypertensive crisis and occurs when blood pressure climbs so high that it may trigger bleeding in the brain. Severe headaches caused by rising blood pressure were also a problem, especially if the person ate tyramine-promoting foods. The early class of MAO inhibitors was found to be so dangerous that it was pulled from the market. After some redesigning, however, MAO inhibitors were reintroduced. They are still considered risky and most doctors only prescribe them in rare instances because they come with serious side effects. They are usually prescribed for chronically depressed individuals who are prone to sleeping or eating excessively.

One side effect of the MOA inhibitor antidepressant drug called phenelzine sulfate (Nardil) is that it can inhibit the action of vitamin B6, which is especially important for maintaining good mental health. Ironically, a deficiency of vitamin B6 is associated with depression. Newer antidepressant medications such as trazodone and maprotiline hydrochloride have fewer side effects than MOA inhibitors; however, they are certainly not without potential drawbacks.

Although the benefits of antidepressant drugs for hundreds of victims of depression should not be overlooked, their hazards and drawbacks should be carefully evaluated. Natural therapies may accomplish the same goal as these medications and should be judiciously investigated. Remember that in the 1960s, these drugs were given a stamp of approval and thought to be relatively safe. MAO inhibitors include:

• isocarboxazid (Marplan)
• phenelzine (Nardil)
• tranylcypromine (Parnate)

SELECTIVE SEROTONIN RE-UPTAKE INHIBITORS (SSRIs)

Selective serotonin re-uptake inhibitors (SSRIs) such as fluoxetine (Prozac), paroxetine (Paxil) and sertraline (Zoloft) make up the most popular line of antidepressants because they are considered safer and have fewer side effects. SSRIs increase brain cells' exposure to serotonin by inhibiting certain processes that actually reduce serotonin levels. As a result, cells stay "bathed" in serotonin longer. Newer versions of these drugs work the same way but with other brain chemicals including serotonin and norepinephrine re-uptake inhibitors (SNRIs) such as nefazodone (Serzone), trazodone (Desyrel) and venlafaxine (Effexor), and dopamine re-uptake inhibitors such as bupropion (Wellbutrin). Even though the SSRIs are considered safer than other types of antidepressant drugs, their use has been associated with side effects like decreased libido, memory loss, insomnia, erratic behavior, agitation, headaches, and mood swings.

Lithium and Other Drugs that Modulate Mood

The medications below are typically used to treat bipolar depression and have a good success rate. They also work as anti-convulsants and are commonly taken by epileptics. Lithium was originally used to treat the dramatic mood swings that accompany manic depression. The drugs typically used for bipolar conditions include lithium (Eskalith, Lithobid), carbamazepine (Epitol, Tegretol), and valproate (Depakene, Depakote).

Some potential side effects include elevated white blood cell count, gum deterioration, liver damage, erratic behavior, and compromised thought patterns. Lithium intake requires close monitoring since too much can cause seizures, coma and in extreme cases, death. Other side effects include metallic taste in the mouth, stomach upsets, diarrhea, tremors, vomiting, and an increase in urine output. Other drugs used less frequently to treat depression include alprazolam (Xanax), methylphenidate (Ritalin), and trazodone (Desyrel).

It is important to note that mood stabilizing drugs such as Depakote are not considered antidepressants; however, they are recommended by some doctors for people who are diagnosed as manic depressive.

Substance P Drugs: New Findings

There is some evidence that a biochemical called substance P plays a profound role in mental health and mood. It was first discovered in 1931, and its action in the body has baffled scientists. Today researchers have discovered that substance P is found in concentrated amounts in the brains of laboratory animals. By blocking this particular chemical, scientists helped some people with migraines, chronic pain and depression. It is now thought that those people with depression who do not respond to traditional treatments may respond to substance P drugs. One clinical trial found that a substance-P blocker worked as well as standard antidepressant drugs in a test group of 210 people. Substance-P

Table 1. A Comparison of Drug Antidepressants

PROZAC
Action:	Inhibits serotonin re-uptake
Advantages:	Low toxicity; used for major depression, as well as mild to moderate depression; nonsedating
Possible Side Effects:	Nausea, loss of appetite, anorgasmia in women, impotence in men, decreased libido, insomnia, nervousness, tremors, tiredness, asthenia, dry mouth, sweating

ZOLOFT
Action:	Works like Prozac
Advantages:	Not as stimulating as Prozac
Possible Side Effects:	Same as Prozac

PAXIL
Action:	Works like Prozac
Advantages:	Not as stimulating as Prozac
Possible Side Effects:	Same as Prozac, plus fatigue

LUVOX
Action:	Works like Prozac
Advantages:	Not as stimulating as Prozac
Possible Side Effects:	Same as Prozac, plus fatigue

EFFEXOR
Action:	Inhibits serotonin and norepinephrine re-uptake
Advantages:	Used for major depression as well as mild to moderate depression

Table 1 (cont.). A Comparison of Drug Antidepressants

Possible Side Effects: Same as Prozac plus nausea, but with less impairment of sexual function than Prozac

TRAZODONE
Action: Inhibits serotonin re-uptake
Advantages: Used for insomnia
Possible Side Effects: Sedation too powerful for mild to moderate depression; severe drowsiness, dizziness, fatigue, nervousness, dry mouth, headache, severe priapism

SERZONE
Action: Inhibits re-uptake of serotonin and norepinephrine
Advantages: Does not interfere with sexual function; is used for anxiety
Possible Side Effects: Too sedating to be useful in mild to moderate depression; headache, sleepiness, dizziness, asthenia, dry mouth, nausea, constipation

WELLBUTRIN
Action: Mildly inhibits re-uptake of serotonin, norepinephrine and dopamine
Advantages: Does not interfere with sexual function; is used for mild, moderate and major depression
Possible Side Effects: Nausea, dry mouth, dizziness, insomnia, agitation, restlessness, anxiety, seizures at high doses

Table 1 (cont.). A Comparison of Drug Antidepressants

TRICYCLICS (Tofranil, Pamelor, Elavil, Sinequan, Ludiomil)

Action:	Inhibits re-uptake of serotonin and norepinephrine
Advantages:	Used for major depression; works rapidly
Possible Side Effects:	Too sedating to be used in mild to moderate depression; fatigue, drowsiness, dry mouth, dizziness, blurred vision, sexual dysfunction, constipation, sweating, heart palpitations, weight gain, urinary retention, cardiac injury at high doses

MAO INHIBITORS (Marplan, Nardil, Parnate)

Action:	Poisons monoamine oxidase, inhibits breakdown of amines
Advantages:	Can work when other drugs fail
Possible Side Effects:	Considered too risky for use in mild to moderate depression; insomnia, dizziness, sexual dysfunction, dangerous with certain foods and over-the-counter drugs

The Overdose Danger: Pharmaceutical vs. Natural

Overdosing on antidepressants can be fatal. Priscilla Slagle, M.D., points out that a number of depressed people will commit suicide by using antidepressants. Moreover, there are countless people who have died from drug-related reactions, whereas death from a nutritional supplement overdose is extremely rare. In fact, statistics tell us that over 100,000 people die annually from prescription drug-related causes as opposed to an average of three from all natural dietary supplements.

blockers may become a new category of antidepressant drugs with fewer side effects than current drug therapies. Large-scale tests to confirm the promise of substance-P drugs are expected to take at least two years before the drugs will be available for prescription.

Drug Therapy: A False Panacea?

Deciding whether or not to begin a conventional drug treatment is not easy. There are definite benefits to such treatments, but nothing comes without risks. And although there is nothing wrong with choosing conventional treatments, it is unfortunate that many people do not know all their options. Conventional treatments can not only bring undesired side effects, they also may not even work, or they may work less effectively over time.

Thomas Szasz once said, "Formerly, when religion was strong and science weak, men mistook magic for medicine; now, when science is strong and religion weak, men mistake medicine for magic." Yes, drug therapy for depression can be effective; however, prescription drugs are grossly overprescribed and often viewed as the only answer. Most doctors are quick to hop on the drug bandwagon, but they rarely tell us that although drugs can provide relief, as many as 30 percent of depressed people fail to respond favorably to even the newest pharmaceuticals available. In fact, many people seem to develop a resistance to the drugs and may need to change drugs or increase dosages to get the desired effect. If you are depressed, you are often forced to weigh the risk of drug side effects against the risk of the disease itself.

If people find it acceptable to experiment with drugs and their dosages to achieve the desired results, why can't they transfer that same attitude to diet, supplementation and other natural methods? Most of us will endlessly fiddle around with potentially harmful medications, yet rarely will we apply this zealous approach to a natural program. The trial-and-error method used by doctors to find the right drug mix can be utilized for natural therapies as well.

Another potential problem with antidepressant drugs is that often their side effects need to be counteracted with other drugs. It's not unusual for doctors to use tranquilizers or sedatives to treat the insomnia that may accompany antidepressant drug therapy— Librium, Valium, Xanax and Ativan are commonly used. In fact, *The American Journal of Psychiatry* revealed that tranquilizers were the only medications used in 643 people surveyed who were being treated in outpatient facilities for depression. Tranquilizers are addictive drugs that may actually worsen depressive symptoms. Becoming dependent on tranquilizers or sleeping pills only further aggravates mood disorders. Most sleeping pills don't provide natural, restful sleep, and tranquilizers rarely cure anything; they just suppress symptoms.

The "Medicate Everything" Approach

Eli Lilly Co. and the producers of Prozac now earn $2.6 billion annually from sales of this drug alone. The Prozac phenomenon, however, has met with growing disillusionment as its side effects continue to take their toll. In addition, it is also estimated that 40 percent of people who take SSRI drugs like Prozac and Zoloft fail to respond. In the not-too-distant future, Prozac may be available as an over-the-counter medication. After all, powerful pain-killing, anti-inflammatory drugs like ibuprofen and Naprosyn used to be available only through prescription but now crowd our grocery store shelves.

Many prominent psychiatrists are concerned that their fellow practitioners have become almost entirely dependent on drug therapy for their patients, preventing them from getting to the real cause of depressive illness. Because chemical treatments are so easy to prescribe, other more beneficial therapies may be ignored. In our country, 80 percent of those diagnosed with depression are quickly given a serotonin-manipulating drug as their first line of treatment. Moreover, these antidepressants are readily dispensed for panic and eating disorders, nicotine addiction, ADHD, and other health problems. The notion that every medicine cabinet in American will contain an antidepressant drug is certainly not far-fetched.

In his book *The Antidepressant Era*, David Healy argues that the notion of one drug for thousands of cases of depression is flawed. He believes, as I do, that depressive illness is a disease of the whole person; therefore, treatment must be tailored according to individual circumstance and need. There is a growing consensus in this country that drugs are taken too freely and prescribed too easily. Because our medicine cabinets are loaded with countless prescription bottles, the risk of drug abuse is extremely high. Undoubtedly, Americans of all ages are using drugs in greater numbers than ever before, and pharmacologic agents designed to elevate moods are at the top of the list. In some cases, drugs are combined with different forms of counseling sessions or psychotherapy. And in some cases, psychotherapy can be used as the sole method of treatment.

Psychotherapy

As mentioned earlier, in some cases of mild depression, short-term psychotherapy (ten to twenty weeks) can be effective. I believe, however, that regardless of the type of depression you have, combining psychotherapy with supplements, light, exercise and other natural treatments makes for a much better mix.

Psychotherapy involves talking it out with a therapist to reveal new perspectives on old problems through a verbal exchange. Behavioral therapies work by assisting you in learning new behaviors that don't result in negative feelings, while helping you leave behind old behaviors that have only served to sabotage your efforts to become content. Interpersonal therapy targets interpersonal relationships that contribute to depression, and cognitive/behavioral therapy works to convert negative thinking and reacting to more positive forms.

ECT (Electroconvulsive Therapy)

Electroconvulsive therapy, or ECT, was once considered barbaric and used only as a last resort, but "shock therapy" (as it is also called) is receiving some new respect. Not too many years ago, doctors tried to wait out depression or use stimulants such as amphetamines to artificially jolt the nervous system. Shock treatments were used only in severe cases, and they earned a bad reputation.

Although it is still considered a drastic form of therapy, ECT has come a long way and according to some doctors, is now used safely and more effectively than drugs. ECT involves attaching electrodes to the scalp and passing a mild current through them, triggering unconsciousness or seizures. This therapy is usually employed in place of drugs and in combination with muscle relaxants and anesthetics to minimize possible side effects.

Today ECT electrical impulses are used in much more restricted dosages after other therapies have failed. In essence, ECT can be effective because it helps "wake up" the brain. In later sections, we'll discuss the fact that the brains of many depressed people seem to be operating on a low-voltage autopilot.

Sending electrical currents through brain cells appears to energize their function, thereby elevating mood. If an individual is at high risk for suicide, has severe anxiety or is acting psychotic, ECT offers quick results and may be the best option in a crisis situation. People who cannot take any medications may be candidates for ECT, although its use is still considered controversial.

Brain Pacemaker

Another possible remedy for a brain that needs to be "revved up" is to use an implant that turns up the wattage. Just like the heart, some scientists have found that if the brain's electrical system is deficient, it may benefit from some artificial stimulation. An ongoing study at fifteen hospitals around the country is looking at stimulating a nerve that runs from the neck into the brain to treat stubborn depression. The new treatment is referred to as "vagus nerve stimulation," and involves sending very small electric shocks into the vagus nerve where the effect is passed up and into the brain. A pilot study found that this therapy achieved very positive results in almost half of thirty depressed individuals who were considered untreatable.

The vagus nerve is a major conduit between the brain and virtually every other body system and organ. The stimulation unit works much like a pacemaker and is implanted into the chest, where electrical impulses are transmitted to the neck. Originally, the device was approved to control epileptic seizures that did not respond to medication. Apparently, an unexpected bonus for these epileptics was that many of them reported feeling happier. I want to mention at this point that magnet therapy is based on a similar notion—that stimulation of the brain from an outside source can alter mood and emotion. The use of magnets for depression is covered in later sections, especially Chapter 21. Although brain pacemakers are not yet available, their existence supports the idea that lethargic brain cell connections are intimately linked to feeling down in the dumps.

CHAPTER 5

Beating Depression Naturally: The Core Protocol

Orthodox medicine has not found an answer to your complaint. However, luckily for you, I happen to be a quack.

RICHTER CARTOON CAPTION

I CHOSE THE above quote to remind all of us that quackery can exist in any profession, no matter how high-minded its practitioners appear to be. Natural medicine has its share of fanatical quacks who pretend to have all the answers to every human ill—for a price. Today, everyone and their dog is trying to get a piece of the alternative medicine "pie," so we must, more than ever before, stay informed with facts rather than fiction.

Ashleigh Brilliant may have been describing the credibility of some natural remedies when he commented, "My sources are unreliable, but their information is fascinating." There's a lot of scuttlebutt floating around out there, and if you don't do your homework, you could very well be throwing your money down the drain. So before you go and spend your hard-earned money on a funny-sounding compound at your local health food store, be convinced that it can really help you.

In the last chapter, we compared natural and conventional medicine, and we reviewed the pros and cons of conventional thera-

pies. In this chapter, we will take a closer look at alternative therapies—what they are, what you can and can't expect from them, and
how they work. In this chapter, you will also be given a basic plan
for treating depression. As you apply the "puzzle-solving
approach" to your depression, you will discover additional factors
that may be contributing to your mood problems. Then, you can
alter or add to the core plan as necessary.

Can Natural Therapies Achieve the Same Results as Drugs?

According to old-time comedian Redd Foxx, health nuts are
going to feel stupid someday, lying in hospitals dying of nothing.
Yes, it's true—no matter how nutritiously we eat and live and
regardless of the number of supplements we take, we will still die.
Granted, we can't prevent death, but we can significantly improve
our living days and even extend them. How we treat our bodies
determines, to a great extent, the quality of our lives.

In the previous chapter we learned that most antidepressants are
designed to elevate levels of specific brain neurotransmitters.
Clearly, if this same effect can be obtained through natural means,
side effects would be minimal. And the fact is, certain naturally
occurring substances can stimulate the same brain processes that
antidepressants can.

Research strongly suggests that through natural methods, we
can achieve the same or similar results as those created by prescription drugs. The key lies in understanding how our bodies
respond to mood changes and knowing what nutritive measures
and supplements to take at the appropriate time. In her book *The
Way Up from Down*, Priscilla Slagle, a medical doctor who suffered
from chronic depression for years, relates how she takes an amino
acid and a B vitamin if she wakes up feeling blue. She writes,

It rarely happens any more these days, but if I ever awaken in the
morning feeling slightly low, I take several tyrosine capsules and put a
few sublingual vitamin B12s under my tongue. Within an hour, my

mood and outlook will have completely improved. I don't have to waste unnecessary time and energy on an unwanted, unneeded state of being, and I experience no side effects whatsoever.

Ideally, all of use would like to recover without drugs. It should be stressed at this point, however, that for some people who become profoundly depressed, antidepressant drugs can be potential life savers. In some severe cases of depression, pharmaceuticals may be the only effective means of control. Keep in mind, however, that certain natural substances such as amino acids, vitamins, enzymes, natural hormones, specific minerals, fatty acids and certain herbs can boost and normalize brain chemistry and function—and unlike antidepressant drugs, they can be infinitely safer. One type of psychiatry that deals with nutrient supplementation is called orthomolecular psychiatry.

Orthomolecular Psychiatry: A Big Term for a Simple Idea

Professor Linus Pauling, who has won the Nobel Prize twice for his work, coined the term "orthomolecular psychiatry," which refers to the treatment of mental disease by providing the most optimal molecular environment for brain cells. He accomplishes this by using certain concentrations of substances normally present in the body. Although most psychiatrists are skeptical of the orthomolecular approach to treating any mental disorder, Dr. Pauling firmly believes that nutrition is crucial to treating the mind and openly condemns the medical establishment's bias against vitamin therapy for mood disorders.

Dr. Pauling cites various studies that conclusively demonstrate the benefits of nutrition for people suffering from schizophrenia. By taking optimum amounts of niacin, ascorbic acid, thiamine, pyridoxine and other nutrients, their mental outlook improved. He states:

In 1970 I was walking along Main Street in the small town of

Cambria, on the coast of California, when a passing car stopped and the driver got out and ran back to me. She said, 'Dr. Pauling, I owe my life to you. I am twenty-six years old. Two years age I was contemplating suicide. I had suffered miserably from schizophrenia for six years. Then I learned about vitamins when someone told me about your paper on orthomolecular psychiatry. The vitamins have saved my life.'

Unfortunately, in their zeal to protect us from quackery, medical doctors have a tendency to throw the baby out with the bath water. There is plenty of scientific evidence that supports using B vitamins, amino acids like tyrosine and 5-HTP, herbs such as St. John's wort, and new natural compounds like SAMe can successfully treat depression. It is difficult for the average person to keep up with these studies however, so I have put together what I like to call the "core protocol" for treating depression naturally. This core protocol is the result of sifting through mountains of data in order to find a basic treatment program for beating depression.

Natural Therapy for Depression:
The Core Compounds

I believe the following compounds hold the most promise as depression therapies. While each of these natural medicines has its own individual merits and drawbacks, some are better than others, depending on your particular needs. So rather than going to the health food store and buying a bottle of each supplement, read on for advice on finding the best combination for you.

How do you know what your needs are and which treatments will benefit those needs? Using the puzzle-solving approach I described in the beginning of this book is a good start. A careful investigation into other possible contributing factors will give you a better idea of what is fueling your depression. After piecing together the reasons behind your depression, look for treatments in this book that are suggested for those contributing factors and then apply a trial-and-error method to figuring out which combinations and dosages work best for you.

Chances are, multiple issues are playing a part in your depressive illness. For this reason, supplemental plans that can be used in addition to the core program laid out in this chapter are described throughout the rest of this book. For example, if your depression is the result of hormonal imbalances, carbohydrate metabolism disorders, bowel disorders, or a low thyroid, you will need to treat these disorders along with your accompanying depression. Your therapeutic strategy should use a combination of the listed supplements as well as other natural medicines designed to treat the underlying physical causes of your mood slump.

I have chosen natural compounds that have the best track record for targeting the cellular pathways and biochemical reactions that have been linked to depression. I based their selection on their complete therapeutic profile and their safety. I am aware, for example, that DHEA has been successfully used to treat depression, but because it is a hormone that may raise the risk of breast, prostate or uterine cancers in some people, I hesitate to recommend it. Other compounds like inositol and phosphatidyl serine may also benefit depression, but studies are not conclusive. In fact, the majority of the nutrients I list are also recommended for optimal health in general.

Note, however, that you should not attempt to stop or reduce any antidepressant or other medication you may be on without the supervision of your doctor. Keep in mind this comment, made by Mark Twain, "Be careful about reading health books. You may die of a misprint." Twain facetiously brings home the point that even natural medicines should be used judiciously and only in appropriate amounts, and they should never be mixed with antidepressant drugs or other medications without the approval of your doctor.

The Core Protocol for Treating Depression

For a more detailed description of each of these compounds and how they work, refer to later chapters. Dietary suggestions and lifestyle changes will also follow in subsequent chapters. (Use a plastic ice tray and keep your total daily supply of supplements in each compartment. This will give you a two-week protocol. Just make sure that each compartment is empty by the evening meal.)

THE BASICS

5-HTP (5-hydroxytryptophan)
Typical dosage: Start with 50 mg daily for a week and then bump up dosage to 100 mg, divided in two doses. Use enteric-coated capsules that can be taken with meals. If your depression is severe, you may want to take 5-HTP and St. John's wort together.
Safety issues: Stomach upset or headaches may occur in some people. Taking 5-HTP with food will help to prevent this effect.

VITAMIN B1
Typical dosage: 100 mg daily

VITAMIN B2
Typical dosage: 50 mg daily

VITAMIN B6
Typical dosage: 50 mg to 100 mg daily

VITAMIN B12
Typical dosage: 800 mcg daily. Use sublingual tablets.

VITAMIN B3
Typical dosage: 400 mg taken twice daily. Use the inositol hexaniacinate form.

FOLIC ACID
Typical dosage: 800 mcg daily

VITAMIN E
Typical dosage: 400 IU daily

VITAMIN C (WITH BIOFLAVONOIDS)
Typical dosage: 1,000 to 4,000 mg daily

GINKGO BILOBA

Typical dosage: 40 mg three times daily. Best if taken before six in the evening. Look for products standardized to contain 24 percent ginkgo flavonone glycosides. Take ginkgo with folic acid and B12 supplements.

OMEGA-3 ESSENTIAL FATTY ACIDS WITH DHA (FROM FISH AND FLAXSEED OILS)

Typical dosage: Take 1 tablespoon of flaxseed oil daily or use capsulized flaxseed oil with a fish oil supplement. Start with two to four capsules daily. Take these with your vitamin E supplement. When buying fish oil, look for products containing 1,000 mg total EFAs that break down to 180 mg of EPA and 120 mg of DHA.

CALCIUM

Typical dosage: 2,000 mg daily; use gluconate or citrate forms for better assimilation. Take with magnesium for optimal results.

MAGNESIUM

Typical dosage: 1,000 mg daily. Take with calcium for best results.

GTF CHROMIUM

Typical dosage: 400 mcg of GTF chromium daily

Add ONE of the following:

SAMe

Typical dosage: 100 to 400 mg daily. Take SAMe in combination with B12 and folic acid supplements to enhance action. Buy only reputable products that guarantee potency and the true inclusion of SAMe. SAMe is particularly good for those suffering from fibromyalgia, rheumatoid arthritis and Parkinson's disease.

Safety issues: Do not take SAMe if you have bipolar depression.

ST. JOHN'S WORT

Typical dosage: 300 mg three times daily of a product with a standardized 0.3 percent hypericin content. Use for a minimum of six to eight weeks. If you find it difficult to sleep, don't take the supplement after six in the evening. Use kava kava root with St. John's wort if insomnia continues to be a problem. If you are not responding to this dosage, try 600 mg three times daily.

Safety issues: Some stomach irritation is possible, and the this herb can increase your sensitivity to sunlight, although it is not likely to happen when taking standard dosages. Photosensitivity is most likely to occur in fair-skinned individuals taking far more than the recommended 900 mg a day. Also, you should not use this herb if you are receiving drug treatment for AIDS. A recent study suggests that St. John's wort may interfere with the action of oral contraceptives and should not be taken prior to surgery due to possible interaction with anesthesia.

NADH (PRINCIPALLY FOR GERIATRIC DEPRESSION)

This form of niacin (nicotinamide adenine dinucleotide) plays a vital role in the energy production of all cells and is thought to boost brain cell metabolism. It is currently used for Alzheimer's disease and seems particularly well suited to older individuals suffering from depression. NADH levels significantly decline with age. NADH supplementation supports the notion that some depression may be due to poor brain cell performance.

Typical dosage: Use 5 to 10 mg once a day on an empty stomach with nine ounces of water. You may want to combine NADH with St. John's wort.

TYROSINE

Typical dosage: Start with 500 mg three times daily and work up to 1,000 mg.

Safety issues: This amino acid may cause agitation and sleeplessness, so don't take it after four in the afternoon. It may also raise blood pressure, so don't use it if you have hypertension.

DLPA (DL-PHENYLALANINE)

Typical dosage: Start with 200 mg twice daily and gradually increase to 400 mg of DLPA before breakfast and another 400 mg dose in the afternoon.

Safety issues: Like tyrosine, DLPA may cause agitation and sleeplessness, so don't take it after four in the afternoon.

A FINAL NOTE

All of these compounds can be used in combination with other treatments in the book that target contributing factors, unless otherwise noted. Of course, it is always a good idea to keep up with the latest research and information about every supplement you decide to take for your depression. Understanding of conventional and alternative treatments in the health community changes daily. Keep in mind, however, as we further discuss possible physical contributors to depression, that the core treatment for depression will be modified according to additional needs and will be listed at the end of each section.

Stellar Brain Foods

In addition to the compounds listed for general depression, there are also a number of foods that are good for mental health and happiness. While whole grain foods, lean meats, and fresh fruits and vegetables provide brain nutrition, fish is particularly beneficial when it comes to preventing depression. The DHA (a fatty acid) content of fish has tremendous value for brain function. Anyone prone to depression should eat fish regularly or take the appropriate supplements.

The following is a list of foods that are particularly beneficial for the brain:

• cold-water fish (i.e. salmon, tuna, sardines)
• fresh blueberries, bananas, oranges
• fresh spinach, collards, mustard greens, asparagus, onions

- garlic
- olive oil
- raw nuts
- soybeans (i.e. tofu, miso)
- swiss cheese
- turkey, liver, eggs
- whole grains

As you may have noticed, the above list covers a wide range of foods. Many of these foods may already be part of your diet, at least to a degree. And don't worry—you won't find long lists of prohibited foods or detailed daily menu plans in this book. I have found that these prescribed eating regimens are difficult to follow and are usually overly restrictive. As a long-term solution, they often predispose us to failure. However, in the next chapter, we will discuss foods and moods, and go into more detail about how to eat in a "brain-friendly" way.

Other Alternative Therapies for Depression

The following is an overview of other therapies that can work to overcome depression. Most of these are detailed in other sections of this book.

- acupuncture
- aromatherapy
- cognitive therapy
- dietary supplements
- electroconvulsive therapy (ECT)
- exercise
- herbal medicine
- magnet therapy
- massage
- meditation
- music
- phototherapy (light)

• psychotherapy
• relaxation response
• support groups
• visualization

    Keep in mind that using any natural therapy takes time and patience. Don't expect to see overnight results. Also, using natural medicine to treat depression works best when it's combined with counseling, meditation and exercise. The success of natural treatments for depression depends on an individual's willingness to learn what and how to eat, their dedication to investigate unique family predispositions, and their openness to supplementation and other alternative treatments. These practices are what the puzzle-solving approach is all about. It relies on your willingness to change your current mind-set and truly embrace the idea that you can get well. Once you change your thinking, you will be able to do the work it takes to solve your depression.

CHAPTER 6

The Mind and Malnutrition

*A light supper, a good night's sleep and a fine morning have often made
a hero of the same man, who by indigestion, a restless night and a
rainy morning, would have proved a coward.*

THE EARL OF CHESTERFIELD

THE HEALTH OF the brain is largely dependent on what you choose
to eat. It's that simple. A study in a 1999 issue of *Public Health
Nutrition* reported the following:

> A deficiency of many vitamins is associated with psychological
> symptoms. In some elderly patients, folate deficiency is associated
> with depression. In four double-blind studies, an improvement in thi-
> amine status was associated with improved mood. Iron deficiency
> anemia is common, particularly in women, and is associated with apa-
> thy, depression and rapid fatigue when exercising.

Consider the fact that in just this study, links are established
between depressed moods and low levels of folic acid, thiamine
and iron in the body. Which prompts the question, are you getting
the nutrients you need to maintain your mental health?

Over the last thirty years, modern technology has changed what
we eat and the way we eat it. Most of our breakfast cereals hardly
resemble the whole grains our grandparents would have eaten for
breakfast, and millions of gallons of sugary and artificially sweet-

ened soft drinks are consumed annually. In fact, we now routinely consume new genetically engineered crop varieties, hormonally fattened beef and poultry, highly processed foods, and a wide variety of food additives and preservatives. Synthetic food substitutes like NutraSweet and synthetic fats are rapidly dominating commercially packaged foods. Furthermore, foods are no longer eaten in season as in past generations. Fruits and vegetables are shipped transcontinentally and are often packed in dry ice or refrigerated for extended periods of time.

In fact, since the 1940s, our body systems have been exposed to thousands of new chemicals that have found their way into not only our foods, but our air and water as well. The recommended daily allowance (RDA) of vitamins and minerals was never set up to deal with the mental and physical stressors that typify our environment. There can be no question that all of these factors play a role in the incidence of mental illness and mood disorders that afflict our generation. This doesn't suggest that other issues aren't involved—it only points out that our low moods may have to do more with deficiencies than with depression. Couple that with the fact that certain circumstances, such as job loss or even the birth of a baby, can trigger brain amine imbalances, and mood disorders become an even bigger problem.

It only stands to reason that if depression can be induced by a malfunction of the brain's biochemistry—whatever the source, it should respond to nutritional modifications (which affect biochemistry). Some cases of depression may even be caused by a lack of certain nutrients or by the misuse of others. One animal study found that nutrient depletion during lactation (nursing) caused significant depression. Another study concluded that even short episodes of early malnutrition for an infant during the suckling period can affect body and brain development, as well as the baby's later susceptibility to depression as an adult.

In fact, in some cases of depression, what's eating at you may be the direct result of what you're eating. Brian Weiss, in a rather old issue of *Psychology Today,* states: "'You are what you eat' may turn out to be as true behaviorally as it is bodily. What you are eating may also be what is eating you, and the relation between a six o'clock dinner and a seven o'clock diatribe may be more causal than casual." Weiss says that the amino acids, which comprise proteins (which compose brain chemicals and determine mood), are all derived from what we choose to eat. He goes on to stress that "the production of neurochemicals in the brain was once thought to be insulated from the meal-to-meal vagaries of amino acid intake. Recent research, however, concludes that what you eat is what you get . . . and perhaps how you act."

To make matters worse, if you have poor eating habits, you may be creating chemical brain patterns that will end up manipulating not only your mood, but also food cravings, weight changes and sleep routines. In fact, your diet and food cravings, weight fluctuations and sleeping schedules should all be analyzed when determining the causes of your depression and how you should treat it. Any or all of these factors can be vital pieces of the depression puzzle, and they should be carefully investigated. But before we go into these factors as a part of our "puzzle-solving" approach, let's explore the physical chemistry behind changes in mood.

Mood Changes as Physical Phenomenon

Most of us are familiar with the links between vitamin C and scurvy, iodine and goiter, calcium and osteoporosis, and iron and anemia. What we're not typically familiar with is research that demonstrates the connection between nutrition and emotional state. If you don't believe that your hunger and how you choose to satisfy that hunger will affect how you behave, think again. It's a scientific fact that hunger can not only cause physical changes in the body, but emotional ones as well.

How many times have you felt grumpy because you've skipped a meal or gone on a carbohydrate-restricted diet? A mood change in cases like these is often the first indication that something is out of kilter with our physiological systems. In fact, scientists at MIT have found that the availability of the amino acids tyrosine and tryptophan in the brain plays a very important role in determining the rate at which four neurotransmitters are produced. Within one hour after a meal, levels of these brain chemicals begin to change as the amounts of tyrosine and tryptophan fluctuate. If you feel depressed for no apparent reason, what you eat may be at fault, and if you are already depressed and you eat poorly, you may intensify your depression.

Natural Health Views Vindicated

What modern medicine is just discovering, natural health practitioners have known for years. In fact, ancient physicians knew that food could either agitate or calm the mind. Modern medicine only needs to relearn what has been known all along—that diet affects individual behavior. In fact, evidence has now vindicated several "nutritional hoaxes" of the past. For instance, many in the medical community now agree that a diet of less fat and sugar, and more fiber, fresh vegetables and whole grains dramatically lowers the risk for some forms of cancer, diabetes, heart disease and colon disorders.

In fact, using diet as treatment is becoming more common. For instance, Johns Hopkins University uses a ketogenic diet to treat pediatric epilepsy. It is a high-fat diet that creates chemically motivated changes in the brain, and in some cases, this treatment has resulted in a complete cure. Unfortunately, because natural treatments and diets are not patentable, you may not find out about these alternatives unless you investigate for yourself.

Ketogenic diets for children with epilepsy have been around for decades, but sadly, only a small percentage of parents are aware of the diet's existence. Instead, as soon as children experience their first seizure, they are immediately put on anticonvulsant drugs and told to get on with their lives. Whereas, something as simple as producing ketones in the body—which is what the ketogenic diet does—can cut the number of and severity of seizures and even cure a significant number of children who suffer from epilepsy if they start early enough. This example illustrates how profoundly our diets can affect the function of our brains. With examples of success like these, why is nutrition still on the back burner for many physicians?

The Neglected Role of Nutrition

Have you ever noticed that after you eat certain foods, you feel like your mood and energy levels crash? Some people feel sudden elation or depression within a few hours of ingesting certain foods or beverages. In response to such phenomena, Dr. Morris Lipton of the University of North Carolina and chairman of the first federally funded conference on nutrition says that the link between food and mood is undeniable. In fact, it is the opinion of several experts that diet is the most frequent cause of depression.

Harvey M. Ross, M.D., believes that many psychiatrists are experiencing a loss of esteem because they refuse to investigate the value of nutritive therapy for mental disorders. He stresses that this lack of objectivity has resulted in the dismissal of a very valuable psychiatric tool. He stresses that it is time for anyone who seeks professional treatment—not only for depression, but also for any other physical or mental disorder—to educate themselves on nutritive options to treating disease.

Research has shown (and continues to show) that a deficiency of just about any nutrient can result in depression. If you eat poorly over an extended period of time, you will inadvertently affect brain neurotransmitters. This is not just true for humans; rats that were put on nutritionally deficient diets became lethargic, indifferent and withdrawn.

Robert Picker, M.D., a California physician, says:

Some people have been brainwashed by traditional medicine into believing that we are getting all the nutrients we need in our average diet, but there are numerous large-scale studies to counter that fallacy. They show there is a large percentage of the American public that is below the Recommended Dietary Allowance (RDA) for many key nutrients, including some of the B vitamins.

In fact, deficiencies of vitamins B1, B6, C and A, along with folic acid, niacin, magnesium, copper, zinc and iron can all cause depression because they influence the production of serotonin and norepinephrine. Again, virtually any nutrient deficiency can result in depression.

Table 1 lists the behavioral effects of eight nutrient deficiencies. Remember these deficiencies when you begin to problem-solve your depression.

Table 1. Abnormal behaviors resulting from vitamin deficiencies.

DEFICIENT VITAMIN	RESULTING BEHAVIOR
Vitamin C	depression, hysteria, hypochondria, lassitude, confusion
Biotin	extreme depression, lassitude, drowsiness
Vitamin B12	depression, psychotic states, irritability, confusion, memory loss, hallucinations, delusions, paranoia, mood swings
Folic acid	depression, apathy, insomnia, irritability, delirium, forgetfulness, psychosis, dementia
Niacin (vitamin B3)	depression, mania, memory deficits, apathy, anxiety, hyperirritability, emotional instability, poor concentration
Pantothenic acid	depression, restlessness, irritability, fatigue, quarrelsomeness
Pyridoxine (vitamin B6)	depression, irritability, nervousness, insomnia, poor dream recall
Thiamin (vitamin B1)	depression, apathy, anxiety, irritability, memory loss, personality changes, emotional instability
Riboflavin (vitamin B2)	depression, insomnia, mental sluggishness

RDA Standards May Not Be Realistic

How much of each nutrient do we need in order to maintain optimal health? To receive the maximum nutritional benefit from our food, our diet would have to consist of several portions of whole grain products; several servings of fresh, raw fruits and vegetables, legumes, nuts, or other protein sources; and adequate, absorbable sources of calcium. Who eats like this every day? I certainly don't. Several studies that analyze diets have discovered that it's common to find at least three to four nutrient deficiencies in our diets, even by RDA standards.

Ideally, we should get what we need from our diet, but in reality, this is rarely the case. Nutrient insufficiencies abound, particularly B vitamin deficiencies, and depression is one of the most prevalent symptoms of a B vitamin deficiency. Moreover, RDA standards may not be designed to take into account the nutrient-depleting effects of pollution and stress. If you assume coming home with bags of fresh fruits and vegetables will provide ample nutrition, think again.

Soil Depletion

Realistically speaking, even if you eat a "balanced" diet that complies with RDA standards, you may still be among the 95 percent of Americans who are deficient in at least one major mineral. Moreover, many people are unaware of soil depletion and its effect on our health. Our mineral-poor earth needs to be taken into consideration when deciding how we will supply ourselves with the nutrients we need.

Experts knew about soil deficiencies as far back as 1936. U.S. Senate Document No. 264 warned Americans that the soils supporting the cultivation of fruits and vegetables were grossly deficient in minerals. If that was the situation seventy years ago, how do you think our soil rates today? And why is this issue so important?

Our health is more dependent on adequate mineral intake than on any other category of nutrients we consume. If you are deficient in vitamins, your body can still make some use of minerals, but when your body lacks minerals, vitamins are useless. Despite this fact, crops are continually harvested and rapidly replanted, which has stripped our soil of the minerals needed to sustain life. In fact, a report from the 1992 Earth Summit in Rio de Janeiro reports that the earth's soil is anemic. In fact, some estimates say that in North America alone, 85 percent of the minerals in farm and range soils have been depleted over the last century.

Fruits, vegetables and grains that are raised on these millions of mineral-deficient acres of land won't supply us with the nutrition we need, regardless of how much of them we eat. In actuality, laboratory tests have found that the harvested foods we eat today are not what they were just a few generations ago. In fact, scientists have labeled at least twenty-six minerals as "bottom line" critical for health maintenance, and even if you are eating a well-balanced diet, you're probably among the 95 percent of Americans who are lacking in at least one of these major minerals!

Forced Harvests and Non-Food Edibles

To make matters worse, we routinely eat crops that have been genetically engineered, and no one really knows how the long-term consumption of such foods will affect our health. In addition, our beef, poultry and pork are rapidly fattened with hormone injections, and the meat is subject to high-tech, chemical processes meant to prevent decay.

Also, unlike our grandparents, we no longer eat fruits and vegetables in season. They are commonly shipped long distances and packed in dry ice or cold storage for extended periods of time. To complicate things, synthetic food substitutes like aspartame and artificial fats like olestra are now in chips and other foods found on our grocery store shelves. (Olestra can rob the body of fat-soluble nutrients like vitamins E, A, K and D.)

Perhaps worst of all, our consumption of caffeine-containing soft drinks inhibits the assimilation of nutrients we do manage to get. For example, the phosphorus found in soda pop causes the body to lose calcium, and white sugar and caffeine can deplete the body of B vitamins and other essential nutrients, as well as cause dehydration. Caffeine does stimulate the release of norepinephrine, which can create a temporary energy surge, but it also inhibits the body's ability to absorb vitamin B1 and causes the loss of magnesium.

The Effect of Hidden Toxins on Your Body's Nutrient Stores

As we talked about earlier, in an ideal world the RDA standards would provide our body with ample nutritional support. Unfortunately, we live in an environment heavily polluted by hundreds of toxic chemicals—most of which remain undetected and are invisible. Many of these poisons actually rob our body of vitamins and minerals. So even if you assume you eat a healthy diet, you may be falling dangerously short of what your body needs to protect itself from hidden toxins, which can affect the levels of nutrients you have in your body. Here are just some of the substances and environmental conditions that destroy B vitamins and various minerals:

- alcohol
- antacids
- anticonvulsants
- barbiturates
- caffeine
- cooking heat
- diuretics
- fever
- heat
- high-protein diets
- mineral oil
- radiation
- sleeping pills
- sugar
- ultraviolet light
- aluminum
- antibiotics
- aspirin
- birth control pills
- chlorine
- cortisone
- estrogen
- food processing
- heavy metals
- laxatives
- oxalic acid
- rancid fats/oils
- stress
- tobacco

The Case for Supplementation

Ultimately, because we do not live in a utopia, it is necessary for us to consider supplementation. The nutritional supplement industry is currently booming, and while taking vitamin and mineral supplements may have raised a few eyebrows among physicians years ago, the practice is well supported by scientific data today. For example, a recent study conducted by scientists at the Harvard School of Public Health reported that taking 100 IU of vitamin E may reduce the development of heart disease by up to 40 percent. I don't know about you, but I don't typically eat the twenty cups of spinach or ten pounds of asparagus required to supply this much vitamin E in the diet. And every month, additional study findings reiterate the need to make sure we get ample amounts of certain nutrients:

- A U.S. study showed that adolescents consumed diets low in several essential vitamins and minerals related to an increased incidence of chronic conditions like ADD, chronic fatigue, depression and even suicide.
- Average calcium consumption in the U.S. and Canada is two-thirds of the RDA level of 800 mg.
- Fifty-nine percent of our calories come from potentially nutrient-poor food sources (e.g. soft drinks, white bread, snack foods).
- The average American receives only half the recommended levels of folic acid.
- Nine out of ten diets contain only marginal amounts of vitamins A, C, B1, B2, B6, chromium, iron, copper and zinc.
- One ambitious, one-day survey of 12,000 people showed that 41 percent ate no fruit, and only 25 percent reported eating a fruit or vegetable that contained vitamin C or A.
- Only one person in five consumes adequate levels of vitamin B6. And as many as 20 percent of people hospitalized for depression are deficient in vitamin B6.
- Seventy-two percent of adult Americans fall short of the RDA recommendation for magnesium.

- The *Journal of Clinical Nutrition* reported that less than 10 percent of those they surveyed ate a balanced diet.
- Up to 80 percent of exercising women and many children have iron-deficient blood.

Interestingly, many health professionals take supplements themselves but don't recommend them to their patients, and data tells us that patients who are well informed take vitamin and mineral supplements anyway. Sadly, the people who don't are the ones who need supplementation the most. A rise in cancer risks alone has been linked to deficiencies in vitamin A, C and E. I believe that the risks are just as significant for mood disorders. Be assured that what you eat or don't eat can affect the way you see yourself and the world around you. Taking the right supplements to protect your health is based on common sense.

Part of any plan for fighting depression should include a vitamin and mineral supplement as well as basic dietary changes. As I said earlier, I don't agree with long, restrictive lists because I think they are counterproductive, but below are general guidelines that you can apply at your own pace and according to your own desires.

Good Eating Tips for Maximum Mood Elevation

I like what George Dennison Prentice said about health and the diet: "What some call health, if purchased by perpetual anxiety about diet, isn't much better than tedious disease." No dietary regimen that is too limiting or too extreme enhances the joy of living. *If you do nothing but eliminate caffeine from your diet, you will have taken a giant step toward better mental and physical health.* Above all, it is important to remember that drastic dietary change will usually fail. If you want changes to your diet to be more long-lasting, change only one aspect at a time. Take it slow! The following are guidelines for effectively revamping your diet:

- Eat a variety of foods to supply all the nutrients your brain requires. Keep meals small and frequent to help your body continually absorb nutrients for better to blood sugar and biochemical levels.

- Add more fish and lean protein to your diet. Also, new varieties of healthy eggs from specially fed chickens are now available. If you don't like fish, take fish oil supplements.
- Begin eating snacks or meals that contain all the food groups.
- Consume organic produce free of pesticides.
- Cut down your intake of white sugar, corn syrup and sweeteners. Instead, eat a diet high in raw fruits, vegetables, whole grains and legumes.
- Don't stay away from foods like raw nuts because of their fat content. Eating healthy snacks comprised of some fat, protein and carbohydrates satisfy us so we don't overeat. A 1999 study published in the *Journal of Clinical Nutrition* found that test subjects ate less carbohydrate foods if they had ingested some fat. Overindulging in fatless carbohydrates can result in fat storage in the body.
- Drink plenty of pure water (at least eight glasses).
- Eat foods rich in fiber and potassium such as beans, sprouts, whole grains, almonds, sunflower seed, lentils, split peas, parsley, blueberries, endive, oats, potatoes with skins, carrots and peaches. Also, eat insoluble fiber on a daily basis (wheat, oat bran, etc.).
- Eat plenty of cabbage, broccoli, brussels sprouts and cauliflower.
- Eat regularly and try to eat at the same time every day to keep your blood sugar levels stable. This will keep your temperament more even and your weight down.
- Incorporate soy foods into your diet. They are full of quality protein and nutritious phytonutrients.
- Combine carbohydrates with protein. The rate at which tryptophan (an amino acid) is converted into serotonin depends on the amount of carbohydrates you eat. In people with faulty carbohydrate digestion, that change is slower than normal, and hunger and overeating persist. Examples: an apple with peanut butter, cottage cheese with a banana, raw almonds with an orange, cheese with a whole-grain cracker, or tuna with whole-grain bread.

• Take nutritional supplements every day.
• Try to use lean meats from animals that have not been hormonally supplemented.
• Use omega-3 fats like olive oil. Avoid using margarines, and use butter sparingly.
• Work on eliminating caffeine, alcohol, nicotine, MSG and unnecessary prescriptions or over-the-counter drugs.
• Your breakfast should be comprised of protein (cottage cheese, raw almonds, eggs, cheese, fish, peanut butter) with whole-grain foods and fresh fruit with the skins on (not fruit juice). Never eat a breakfast made up of only carbohydrate foods, even if they are whole-grain. Protein and fats help to delay the conversion of carbohydrates to blood sugar. If you only eat carbohydrates, you will get abnormally hungry around midmorning and crave sugars and starches; you may also experience a mood slump.

How To Select Quality Nutritional Supplements

Although we may make every attempt to optimize our eating habits, sometimes we fall short of the ideal diet. Consequently, dietary supplements can help us make up the difference. The following provide sound guidelines for choosing the supplements that will best help you.

• All supplements, including herbs, are not created equal. Look for "clinically tested" and "proven bioavailability" on supplement labels. Reputable companies have their own research and development departments with qualified professionals.
• Avoid products that contain sugar, starch, salt, coal tars, yeast, corn, milk or artificial colorings or flavorings.
• Avoid time-released supplements. There is some evidence that they don't work as well as standard vitamin and minerals.
• Be wary of big, hard, "horse" pills in compressed tablets that may not completely dissolve. There is substantial evidence indicating that such tablets often pass through the digestive and eliminatory tracts largely undigested. (I recently conducted a vinegar test on

some of these and found that very little of the pill dissolved, even after 24 hours.)

- Buy minerals that have been "chelated." Amino acids should be "free form."
- Calcium gluconate, aspartate, lactate, citrate or glutarate are considered the most absorbable kinds of calcium. I personally like the calcium citrate variety.
- Choose lactobacillus acidophilus that contains bifidobacteria and check the expiration date often.
- Don't take any fat-soluble vitamins with a fiber supplement or their potency will be impaired.
- Each day, take vitamin and mineral supplements with your meals for better digestibility. Also, take your supplements at the same time each day.
- Good protein sources come from soy or whey.
- GTF chromium seems to have a better safety profile than picolinate forms.
- If you need extra zinc, use picolinate varieties or zinc lozenges.
- Iron (ferrous gluconate) is more absorbable than sulfate.
- Look for combination vitamin and mineral supplements that contain biotin, which some companies skimp on because of expense.
- Purchase broad-spectrum antioxidants that contain beta-carotene, selenium, vitamin E, lipoic acid, vitamin C and grape-seed extract if possible.
- Take an amino acid supplement on an empty stomach with a little fruit juice.
- Try to buy vitamin E, selenium and chromium supplements that come from natural sources.
- Use an egg carton or plastic ice tray to put in a two-week supply of what you need, and make sure it is empty by the end of the day.
- Vitamin B12 is destroyed during digestion, so buy it in a sublingual capsule.

CHAPTER 7

Sugar and Serotonin

What you eat can make you a mellow fellow, a sad lad, or a wild child.
UNKNOWN

NOT LONG AGO, this scene was all too common in my life: while working at the computer, I get an intense craving for something sweet and head off to the kitchen to polish off a bag of oatmeal cookies, which I wash down with glass of root beer, juice or other sugar-laden drink. As one can imagine, the results of this continual sugar-binging were nothing less than disastrous. Keep in mind that the average American eats over 125 pounds of white sugar every year. It has been estimated that sugar makes up 25 percent of our daily calorie intake, with soft drinks topping the list. Americans also eat an average of fifteen quarts of ice cream per person per year.

As a society, we have become obsessed with sugar, not fully recognizing what excessive sugar consumption does not only to the body, but also the mind. Sugar is a powerful substance that can have druglike effects, and it is considered addictive by a number of nutritional experts. In fact, excess amounts of sugar can be toxic. Significant amounts of B vitamins are required to metabolize and detoxify ingested sugar. Moreover, when you overload the body with sugar, you can inhibit the assimilation of nutrients from other foods. Nevertheless, our diets are loaded with sugar—hidden and added—from our first bowl of candy-sweet, cold cereal to our daily jumbo-sized soda, to our excessive consumption of chips, candy bars and pastries.

Cutting down our sugar consumption is probably one of the best things that we can do for our overall health—physical and mental. It can also be one of the hardest things to accomplish. We will discuss the reasons for this later in the chapter. Regardless of how difficult it can be to curb our sugar consumption, our bodies were not designed to cope with the high quantity of sugar we routinely consume. Too much sugar can generate a type of nutrient malnutrition that, according to a number of experts, can affect the way we behave. It is important that we pay attention to how much sugar we are including in our diet. Among other things, too much sugar can predispose us to yeast infections, aggravate some types of arthritis and asthma, cause tooth decay, elevate blood fats, and make us obese or diabetic.

Ultimately, you may discover that your sugar intake is a large piece in your depression puzzle because sugar so directly affects brain chemistry (as well as countless other things). This chapter will help you analyze the effects of sugar on your body and your mind. As you read this section, carefully evaluate your own sugar consumption habits and how they may be linked to your moods. Identifying your body's relationship to sugar will help you construct a plan to fight your depression.

Why Do We Crave Sugar if It Is So Bad For Us?

It's hard to ignore a bad sweet tooth, and the question remains, if sugar is so bad for us, why do some of us crave it so intensely? The answer is simple. Sugar gives us a quick infusion of energy and can even temporarily lift our spirits, which can also explain, at least in part, why it can be addictive. The effects of sugar are particularly appealing to those of us who are fatigued or feeling blue.

Of course, our bodies need a certain amount of glucose, but be assured that they were never designed for twentieth century life where we have instant access to unlimited amounts of sugar. In fact, most of our children don't think of sugary foods as special treats anymore, and for some of them, sugar is a food staple. Twenty years ago, candy was available to most American children only at Christmas, Halloween or other special events. A fresh orange in the Christmas stocking was considered a wonderful and sweet delicacy. Today, however, our homes, schools and workplaces are teeming with candy, cookies, cakes, highly sweetened cold cereal and beverages. What's so insidious about consuming sugar? The more you eat, the more you want.

Sugar and Behavior

Blood sugar surges and dips can play a major role in determining whether we are agreeable or cantankerous. Excess sugar and starch are difficult for our bodies to tolerate, and for some of us, eating them can make us act rather intolerably as well. Have you ever been around someone who is prone to mood swings characterized by violent verbal attacks and sudden irritability? Normal people don't go on an unprovoked rampage. This type of volatile behavior is typical of some people who crave sugar, eat it and then experience erratic behavior.

As you apply the puzzle-solving approach to your diet, and in particular, your sugar consumption, it is important that you notice your behavior before and after you eat foods. Be aware of your mood and energy levels as they relate to sugar consumption. Does your behavior change after eating sugar? What characterizes your mood when you begin to crave a sugary item? Remember, too, that your sugar cravings may be related to drops in brain amine levels that cause you to feel lethargic and emotionally shot.

Sugar Can Be Hazardous to Your State of Mind

The amino acids tryptophan and phenylalanine have to compete with sugar for absorption in the intestines. They are also the building blocks for the brain chemicals that sustain a good mood. For this reason, nutritionists have long advised against eating protein and sugar at the same time, since protein supplies our bodies with amino acids. Consuming sugar and protein at the same time can inhibit absorption of the amino acids you need for a healthy mood.

What's worse, we can actually become dependent on sugar. In his book *Sugar Blues,* William Dufty writes, "The difference between sugar addiction and narcotic addiction is largely one of degree." Perhaps it would be more accurate to refer to sugar as a substance that has a druglike effect on the body. In and of itself, a moderate amount of sugar consumed now and then may be perfectly harmless to most people. The potential problem with eating a little sugar, however, is that it stimulates our appetite for more sugar. I know that if I eat a lot of sweets over the holidays, I find it very difficult to taper off afterwards. January is a particularly bad month for me, due in part to the residual effects of December feasting and the dark, drab winter weather. Keep in mind also that if you abruptly cut off your sweet supply, you can feel fatigued, irritable, headachy and depressed. These are signs of withdrawal, further supporting the idea that sugar is addictive.

Brain Chemistry and Sugar's Vicious Cycle

How is sugar addictive? You probably know that eating refined sugars and carbohydrates raises blood insulin levels, but you may not know that this process also raises serotonin levels in the brain. As a result, after eating sugar you may feel a short-lived mood elevation. The fact that so many of us reach for a candy bar or bag of chips during our afternoon slump at the office illustrates the quick energy and mood boost sugar can provide. One Colorado internist comments:

> People who are chronically stressed and are on a roller coaster of blood sugar going up and down are especially prone to dips in energy at certain times of day. Their adrenals are not functioning optimally, and when they hit a real low point, they want sugar. It usually happens in mid-afternoon when the adrenal glands are at their lowest level of

functioning. I have them take glutamine at that point because it helps to regulate the glucose in the brain.

Because of the effect of sugar on serotonin, it is now thought that if we continually eat excessive amounts of sugar or carbohydrates, the brain will no longer produce or utilize serotonin the way it should. In other words, excessively high sugar and insulin levels can disrupt the way serotonin is synthesized and used. As a result, brain cells may suffer from inadequate serotonin stimulation. Consequently, you may experience mood slumps that prompt the consumption of more sugar to counteract the effect, and the cycle marches on.

Some experts have pointed out that this cycle of sugar addiction is similar to one seen with a brain chemical called dopamine and the use of alcoholic drinks. Drinking alcohol causes an initial surge of dopamine in the brain, which makes you feel better, but in time not only does this effect wear off, but the natural dopamine-producing processes in the brain become impaired, resulting in a lack of dopamine. When dopamine dips, so does your mood, which prompts even more drinking in an attempt to feel okay again.

The same phenomenon can happen with sugar. Like alcohol, the effect of sugar on increased energy and mood is temporary and quickly wears off. The effect of the insulin, however, lasts longer and contributes to depression and feelings of fatigue, which stimulates the consumption of more sugar. Excessive carbohydrate or sugar cravings pose a particularly challenging problem for certain individuals who may suffer from carbohydrate metabolism disorders. For these people, food and mood are intimately linked.

The Wurtman Study: Linking Food and Mood

Richard Wurtman, M.D., and Judith Wurtman, Ph.D., professors at the Massachusetts Institute of Technology (MIT), were the first to link food with mood when they found that the sugar and starch in carbohydrate foods boosted serotonin levels. Their studies have profoundly changed the way we look at food and brain function. They were able to link serotonin and other neurotransmitters to behavior, mood and food cravings. For instance, they noted that eating carbohydrate-rich foods (breads, cereals, pasta, fruits and starchy vegetables such as potatoes, winter squash, or corn) increased serotonin levels, which resulted in heightened relaxation. On the other hand, eating high-protein foods such as cottage cheese, beans, peas, nuts and soy had the opposite effect. Apparently, high-protein foods prompt the body to release chemicals that make you feel more alert and energetic. According to Dr. Judith Wurtman, who has done extensive research in this field, there are three types of triggers that cause quick and dramatic changes in brain activity:

• Caffeine acts as a brain stimulant and a temporary energy source.
• Carbohydrates (whole grains, vegetables, sugars) promote calm, reduce anxiety and stress and help to focus the mind.
• Proteins (animal foods, legumes) help to promote the stimulation of the brain and produce energy.

It is also important to note that new data tells us that the fats we choose to eat also influence our brain chemistry; this is discussed more fully in other sections of the book. More than any other study, the Wurtman findings dramatically illustrate that the foods we choose to eat influence our behavior and emotional well being. Judith Wurtman points out that when we make poor food choices, not only do we put our physical health in jeopardy, but we impact our emotional landscape as well. She stresses that what we eat can contribute to or take away from our feelings of self-worth and confidence. Her ideas are based on the holistic notion that the human body cannot be treated in parts and that all of its facets (physical, emotional and spiritual) react to our lifestyle choices. This study is particularly relevant to discussions of depression and underpins the entire thrust of this book.

Serotonin Levels, Carbohydrate Cravings and Depression

If you find yourself craving snacks like cookies or chips on a consistent basis and if you suffer from depression, your mood fluctuations may be related to how your serotonin levels are affected by your blood sugar levels. One of the most fascinating things to come out of the Wurtman study is the idea that *people who excessively crave carbohydrates also show a high susceptibility to clinical depression.* In other words, if you have a tendency to crave carbohydrate snacks, you may not be eating just to satisfy hunger. You may crave these snacks to boost your mood. Typically, do you eat just one or two cookies if you occasionally crave something sweet, or do you find yourself eating cookie after cookie until the whole package is gone? If you do the latter, you may be a victim of a carbohydrate-related mood disorder.

In one study, people who snacked excessively on carbohydrates were asked why they continually ate foods they knew would pack on the weight. They responded that they ate to combat tension, feelings of anxiety or mental fatigue. Eating several cookies or potato chips gave them a feeling of calmness and well being. Further research at MIT has shown that some obese people use sugar or carbohydrates as a type of sedative to maintain this sense of contentment. Unfortunately, when sugar levels dropped, their feelings of anxiety and depression returned.

Food as an Antidepressant

An additional study done at MIT gave psychological tests to forty-six volunteers before and after they ate a meal rich in carbohydrates. Those who were considered habitual carbohydrate cravers were significantly less depressed after eating the food. On the other hand, noncravers became tired and sleepy. This study tells us that appetite fluctuations may be motivated by mood disorders. It also suggests that for some people, food cravings are the body's way of trying to elevate certain neurotransmitters in the brain that create sensations of security and contentment. In so doing, some people find themselves continually craving and snacking, a phenomenon which is not always related to true hunger. Frequently, people who fall into this category will gain weight due to the caloric nature of most carbohydrate snacks, which only serves to further decrease their feelings of self worth.

Remember that the production of serotonin, which is made from tryptophan, depends on carbohydrate intake. Blood levels of tryptophan increase when carbohydrates are consumed. Tryptophan crosses the blood-brain barrier and is converted into serotonin. The rate of this conversion is dependent on the proportion of carbohydrates eaten. Carbohydrates stimulate the production of insulin, which permits the uptake of most amino acids into cells. Studies indicate that when brain levels of serotonin decrease, some people begin to crave carbohydrates. The study also points out that with some people who have trouble with mood swings or even PMS, the brain fails to respond as it should when starchy snacks are eaten, therefore the craving persists and overeating occurs.

Insulin, Appetite and Blood Sugar

One of the most powerful influences on appetite is our blood sugar level. The more we stabilize blood sugar and insulin levels, the more we can control our carbohydrate cravings. In his book *The Zone*, Barry Sears addresses what happens when we reach for starchy or sweet snacks to satisfy our hunger: "In desperation, your brain tells you that bag of corn chips looks very inviting. While eating the corn chips (or Oreo cookies) does supply an immediate source of carbohydrates for the brain, it simply restarts the vicious circle of raised insulin and diminished glucagon [stored sugar]." To make matters worse, if we suffer from hypoglycemia, our blood sugar levels plunge too low and we experience intense hunger for something sweet or fattening. This effect can cause even the most disciplined dieter to attack the potato chip bag or tray of brownies, so the vicious cycle repeats itself.

After insulin has contributed to carbohydrate storage instead of creating a feeling of satisfaction, it signals the brain to stimulate the appetite so you want to snack again and again. Experts believe that this constant glut of carbohydrate consumption can result in the oversecretion of insulin causing even lower blood sugar levels and more intense periods of hunger. These cravings get worse as time goes by. This explains why so many of us get hungry one or two hours after eating a high-carbohydrate meal. This may also explain why we experience lows and highs throughout the day. Some of us overreact biologically and emotionally when we eat foods that quickly raise our blood sugar. Technically, when your blood sugar levels continually plummet after eating sugars or carbohydrates due to an excessive insulin response, you may have what some experts call hypoglycemia.

Hypoglycemia: Fact or Fiction?

The brain is highly dependent on glucose (blood sugar) for its energy source. When blood sugar levels drop, hormones go into action. It is the release of adrenaline that causes the "sugar shakes"—sweating, tremors, hunger and weakness. These symptoms usually accompany a sudden and dramatic drop in blood sugar. Keep in mind that if your blood sugar levels decrease gradually, you may not recognize your symptoms as those of hypoglycemia. You may feel dizzy, confused, clouded and emotionally unstable without any visible tremors. If you have these episodes on a regular basis, you may be suffering from hypoglycemia.

Because hypoglycemia is not really understood by the medical community, it is often brushed off as a bogus malady. One reason for this denial is the inadequacies of the five-hour glucose tolerance test (GTT) as an effective diagnostic tool. I know that I have hypoglycemia. If I eat a bowl of sugared cold cereal, I go into some serious tremors approximately two hours later. Many cold cereals contain such highly refined sugars that they cause blood sugar levels to shoot up quickly. In some people, the pancreas tries to compensate with excess insulin, which only ends up pushing down those blood sugar levels to extreme lows. When blood sugar gets this low, our brain is profoundly influenced.

In addition, new studies are revealing that some psychological disorders are directly linked with disturbed glucose utilization in brain cells. One study, in particular, showed that depressed people have overall lower glucose metabolism, which affects primarily the front and left sections of the brain and therefore also impacts behavior and mood.

In fact, in some circles, hypoglycemia is considered the most common cause of depression. In a study of 500 people with hypoglycemia, 75 percent were found to be suffering from significant depression. Harvey Ross, M.D., believes that hypoglycemia should always be considered whenever a patient complains of depression. Your doctor can order a glucose tolerance test, but keep in mind that this test is not always accurate. Dr. David R. Hawkins, medical director of the North Nassau Mental Health Center, has performed five-hour glucose tests which were perfectly normal for the first three hours and then showed a dramatic drop during the fourth hour. Dr. Ross points out that 90 percent of treatable hypoglycemia can be missed.

What is normal for one person may not be for another. He goes on to say that sometimes tests come back normal, but symptoms of hypoglycemia persist. He cautions against relying solely on test numbers. Determining the level at which symptoms of hypoglycemia will occur is extremely difficult and varies with each individual. He points out that recent research suggests that 50 mg/dl blood is too high a reading.

Normal blood sugar ranges in the 60 to 100 mg/dl blood. When blood sugar drops below 50 mg/dl, adrenaline is secreted to prompt the release of stored sugar from the liver. This mechanism that compensates for low blood sugar is also associated with a number of individual-specific symptoms that can include everything from short tempers to fainting. Interestingly, PMS can be commonly accompanied by hypoglycemic episodes suggesting that estrogen and progesterone impact the way we crave and process sugar. Ultimately, it is your individual biochemistry that determines whether you are prone to hypoglycemia or not, wherein heredity also plays a role.

Is Hypoglycemia Contributing to Your Depression?

Examining your eating habits—what you eat, when you eat it and what happens during the following hours—may be more informative than any diagnostic lab test. Anyone who feels depressed in combination with crying spells, anxiety, temper outbursts, headaches or apprehension should suspect low blood sugar levels. In addition, you need to examine your genetic history—hypoglycemia runs in families.

Some studies have shown that up to 77 percent of people who experience low blood sugar suffer from depression. Unquestionably, people who suffer from hypoglycemia are strongly predisposed to depression. Oscar Janiger, M.D., in his book *A Different Kind of Healing,* talks about one of his patients who had been treated for depression with drugs and psychotherapy for ten years. After reading a magazine article, she announced to him that she had been misdiagnosed and really should have been treated for low blood sugar. Naturally, Dr. Janiger was skeptical but reluctantly administered a blood glucose test that revealed she did indeed suffer from hypoglycemia.

Anyone who consistently fights depression that cannot be connected with any other factors should investigate the possibility that they have low blood sugar. Even if there are other contributing factors, low blood sugar may be part of the puzzle. And the solution is relatively simple. Switching your diet from one high in refined carbohydrates to one comprised of protein and complex carbohydrates could mean the difference between a dysfunctional life and a rich one. People who have suffered with hypoglycemic mood disorders and have learned to eat differently frequently comment that they feel like they're off of the emotional seesaw.

One such person described himself as "incredibly depressed." He frequently missed work and had great difficulty just dragging him-

Table 1. Symptoms of hypoglycemia.

Symptoms of hypoglycemia can vary from person to person. Anxiety attacks are often linked with the disorder, as well as apathy, paranoia, phobias, delusions, confusion and depression. The following symptoms can result from hypoglycemia. Notice how many of these symptoms are similar to those listed for classic depression.

- allergies
- anxiety or excessive worrying
- crying spells
- depression
- digestive disturbances
- drowsiness
- excessive sighing or yawning
- exhaustion
- faintness or dizziness
- fluctuating moods
- forgetfulness
- headaches
- heart palpitations
- hot flashes
- impotence
- indecisiveness
- insomnia
- intense craving for sweets
- irritability
- mental confusion
- muscle pains or leg cramps
- nervousness
- numbness
- outbursts
- rage
- social withdrawal
- tremors or cold sweats
- uncontrolled appetite
- vertigo

Typically, if you suffer from hypoglycemia, you will feel good right after you eat, and then your mood and physical status will deteriorate two to six hours after. If you suspect that you might suffer from low blood sugar, examine your dietary history carefully. Do your have a family history of diabetes, alcoholism or low blood sugar? Do you crave carbohydrates on a consistent basis? Do you feel at your worst in the morning? If you have several of the symptoms listed above, you may wish to read *Fighting Depression* by Harvey Ross, M.D., which delineates in detail the dietary strategy necessary to control this disorder.

self out of bed in the morning. Morning meant feeling lousy. He typically woke up with a headache and felt nauseated. This man was subsequently tested for glucose intolerance. He told his present doctor that he suspected he had hypoglycemia but had received no support from his previous physician. In fact, not one of the doctors he had visited asked him about his dietary habits, and certainly none of them suggested that his diet may be linked to his depression. This man had practically lived on soft drinks and candy bars. Let me stress here that caffeine and sugar are referred to as the nutritional precursors of depression by some experts. This man was subsequently placed on a low-carbohydrate diet of whole grains and low-fat meats and fish, along with supplements of vitamins B6 and B12, folic acids, tryptophan and pantothenic acid. Within a month, he felt entirely better and his depression disappeared.

Hypoglycemic depression is usually typified by low energy levels without any event that would normally accompany the "blues." People who suffer from this kind of depression will often comment that they have a good life and should be happy, but they feel downcast and glum.

To Eat or Not to Eat: Food Choices to Prevent Sugar Blues

In several cases of depression, when foods are eliminated from the diet that cause severe blood sugar swings, patients are able to control their depression even when years of psychotherapy and drugs failed them. Sugar and caffeine should be the first to go, or at least be carefully managed.

The elimination of foods such as candy, soda pop, doughnuts and other sugary pastries, sugared cold cereals and cookies can really make a difference in blood-sugar motivated depression. These foods quickly raise blood glucose levels and initiate a rush of insulin, which brings those levels way down. Dr. August F. Daro, an obstetrician/gynecologist in Chicago says, "A lot of depressed people don't eat well . . . perhaps they'll have a cup of coffee and a sweet roll for breakfast. I make sure they eat three good meals every day. A good diet has to be the foundation of the nutritional treatment of depression."

It is also interesting to learn that nocturnal hypoglycemia, which refers to a low nighttime blood sugar level, can also promote insomnia. As mentioned earlier, when blood sugar drops, adrenaline is released that stimulates the brain and signals to the body that it is time to eat. If you eat a piece of cheese with whole grain snack thirty minutes before going to bed, you can avoid this scenario. Complex carbohydrates that take time to break down can help to sustain normal blood sugar levels throughout the night. In addition, as we have discussed, these types of foods increase serotonin levels in the brain that helps promote sleep. Whatever you do, don't eat highly refined, sugary snacks before going to bed. Eating a big bowl of sugar frosted flakes before you go to bed is one of the worst things you can do.

Keep in mind also that when some people stop eating white sugar and refined carbohydrates, they may feel worse at first due to sugar withdrawal, and mood swings may still be a problem. If this is the case, Dr. Ross suggests eating wholesome snacks high in protein and complex carbohydrates every two hours to prevent the blood sugar from dropping. He also recommends adding B-complex vitamins to the diet.

In summary then, if you suspect that you are hypoglycemic and suffer from depression, concentrate on adding more of these foods into your diet:

• eggs
• fish
• low-carbohydrate vegetables (i.e. beet greens, cucumbers, lettuce, radishes, asparagus, broccoli, cabbage, cauliflower, mushrooms, onions, peppers, tomatoes, squash, spinach, zucchini)
• nuts and seeds
• unsweetened yogurt
• vegetable juices
• white meats
• whole grains (including pasta)

It's important to note that fruits should be limited to two or three servings per day and should be eaten as part of a meal rather than a separate snack. Recommended fruits include berries, cantaloupe, coconut, muskmelon, cranberries, casaba melon and lemons/limes.

FOODS TO AVOID

Just as there are foods that should be emphasized to combat low blood sugar, there are also foods that should be avoided or eliminated altogether to improve a hypoglycemic state. These include the following:

• alcohol
• artificial sweeteners
• caffeine
• high-fat, empty calorie foods (e.g., doughnuts, soft drinks)
• processed or enriched foods (white flour and sugar)
• quick cooking grains
• undiluted fruit juices

The Glycemic Index

Glycemic rating systems are useful because they measure how fast a particular food is likely to raise your blood sugar. Remember that the quicker a food is metabolized and enters the bloodstream, the more excessive insulin response can be. For example, most sweetened cold cereals have a tendency to spike our blood sugar and can cause hypoglycemic effects due to an exaggerated insulin response. Table 2 provides an index based on the glucose content of food, which is absorbed quickly. Glucose is given a value of 100 and other carbohydrate foods have been assigned a value as it relates to glucose. The carbohydrates that are metabolized faster and raise blood sugar quicker have higher number values. These numbers may not be the same as ones found on other glycemic tables; they were supplied by the Diabetes Mall for use by diabet-

Table 2. The glycemic index.

BEANS
baby lima 32
baked 43
black 30
brown 38
butter 31
chickpeas 33
kidney 27
navy 38
pinto 42
red lentils 27
split peas 32
soy 18

BREADS
bagel 72
Kaiser roll 73
pita 57
pumpernickel 49
rye 64
rye, whole 50
white 72
whole wheat 72
waffles 76

CEREALS
All Bran 44
Bran Chex 58
Cheerios 74
corn bran 75
Corn Chex 83

cornflakes 83
Cream of Wheat 66
Crispix 87
Grapenuts 67
Grapenuts Flakes 80
Life 66
Muesli 60
NutriGrain 66
oatmeal 53
oatmeal 1 min 66
puffed wheat 74
puffed rice 90
rice bran 19
Rice Chex 89
Rice Krispies 82
Shredded Wheat 69
Special K 54
Team 82
Total 76

COOKIES/CRACKERS
oatmeal 55
shortbread 64
Vanilla Wafers 77
Kavli Norwegian 71
rye 63
saltine 72

DESSERTS
angel food cake 67
bran muffin 60

Table 2 (cont.). The glycemic index.

Danish 59
fruit bread 47
pound cake 54
sponge cake 46

FRUIT
apple 38
apricot, canned 64
apricot, dried 30
banana 62
banana, unripe 30
cherries 22
fruit cocktail 55
grapefruit 25
grapes 43
kiwi 52
mango 55
orange 43
pear 36
pineapple 66
plum 24
raisins 64
strawberries 32
watermelon 72

GRAINS
barley 22
brown rice 59
buckwheat 54
bulgar 47
chickpeas 36
cornmeal 68

hominy 40
millet 75
rice, instant 91
rice, parboiled 47
rye 34
sweet corn 55
whole wheat 41
white rice 88
white rice, high amylose 59

JUICES
apple 41
grapefruit 48
orange 55
pineapple 46

MILK PRODUCTS
chocolate milk 34
ice cream 50
milk 34
yogurt 38

PASTA
brown rice pasta 92
linguine, durum 50
macaroni 46
macaroni & cheese 64
spaghetti 40
spag. prot. enrich. 28
vermicelli 35
vermicelli, rice 58

Courtesy of the Diabetes Mall

ics. Variables such as fruit ripeness, fat content and fiber content all determine how quickly sugars are absorbed. Your own fitness and exercise habits also affect how quickly sugars are absorbed.

As we mentioned, when you first start to eat this way, you will probably feel lousy. You may get weak, dizzy, nauseous and even more depressed. This is particularly true if you have been eating a diet high in white sugar and fat, but if you give the diet a chance, you will feel a dramatic improvement in mood and physical well-being. Your body takes time to adjust; beneficial results won't be seen overnight. You will still have good days and bad days, but in time, you'll notice less variation in your moods as your body adjusts. Within three to five weeks, you should be able to think more clearly, wake easier and generally feel good about life. Remember that nutritional treatments for depression require the teamwork of a revised diet and supplementation. Yes, it does take time, but it certainly is worth the effort.

A Note on Artificial Sweeteners

Switching to artificial sweeteners to help you control your blood sugar may not be a good idea. Although they have received the FDA stamp of approval, compounds like aspartame and saccharin are routinely consumed with little thought to their health risks. Andrew Weil, M.D., in his book *Natural Health, Natural Medicine,* writes:

More worrisome than preservatives are artificial sweeteners. Saccharin, a known carcinogen, should be avoided. Cyclamates, banned some years ago for suspected carcinogenicity, are not being reconsidered for use in food. They taste better than saccharin but cause diarrhea in some people. Avoid them too. Recently, aspartame (NutraSweet) has become enormously popular. The manufacturer portrays it as a gift from nature, but, although the two component amino acids occur in nature, aspartame itself does not. Like all artificial sweeteners, aspartame has a peculiar taste. Because I have seen a number of patients, mostly women, who report headaches from this substance, I don't regard it as free from toxicity. Women also find that aspartame aggravates PMS (premenstrual syndrome). I think you are better off using moderate amounts of sugar than consuming any artificial sweeteners on a regular basis.

While thousands of Americans continue to consume aspartame in unprecedented amounts, controversy surrounding its safety lingers. Dr. Richard Wurtman of the Massachusetts Institute of Technology (MIT) and author of some of the studies I've talked about has reported that abnormal concentrations of neurotransmitters developed when he fed laboratory animals large doses of aspartame. He believes that the phenylalanine content of the sweetener actually manipulates and alters certain brain chemicals that could initiate behavioral changes and even seizures. He suggests that while small quantities of aspartame may be safe, the cumulative effects of the compound, particularly if consumed with high-carbohydrate, low-protein snacks, could be serious.

Aspartame has been marketed as a safe substance for the general public except for those few individuals who suffer from PKU (phenylketonuria), a relatively rare disorder. Most consumers assume that aspartame is a perfectly benign compound and use it liberally. It is, in fact, comprised of phenylalanine, aspartic acid and methanol (wood alcohol). As previously mentioned, various side effects have been associated with the ingestion of aspartame—migraines, memory loss, slurred speech, dizziness, stomach pain and even seizures.

In addition, because aspartame contains chemicals that affect brain cell function, significant questions have been raised concerning its link to increased incidence of brain tumors. Acesulfame K, another artificial sweetener on the market, has also been linked to cancer by the Center for Science in the Public Interest. In spite of these findings, these sweeteners have been approved by the FDA and are recognized as safe.

Using Stevia as a Sugar Substitute

Stevia may offer the answer for anyone wanting a safe sweetener. It has all the benefits of artificial sweeteners and none of the drawbacks. Stevia can be added to a variety of foods to make them "sweet" without adding calories or impacting the pancreas or adrenal glands. It can help to satisfy carbohydrate cravings without interfering with blood sugar levels or adding extra pounds. Using stevia to create "treats" for children is also another excellent way to avoid weight gain, tooth decay and possible hyperactivity. While it may take some getting used to initially, stevia products are becoming easier to measure and are better tasting.

When the whole-leaf extract or powdered forms of stevia come in contact with the taste buds, the resulting taste can be described as a combination of sweet with a slight licorice-like and transient bitter flavor. If stevia is used correctly with hot water or other liquid, both of these undesirable flavors will disappear. Currently, researchers are working on a new extraction process that will preserve stevia's sweetening potency while minimizing any aftertaste associated with the herb.

Supplement Game Plan for Carbohydrate Metabolism Disorders (use with Core Protocol)

HIGH-FIBER SUPPLEMENT
Background information: Fiber has a good track record for blood sugar control. The complex-carbohydrates structure of fiber can reduce the speed at which sugar enters the blood stream. Psyllium is especially good for diabetics. It can reduce glucose elevation by 31 percent.

Typical dosage: Take as directed, using products designed to be mixed with water or juice first thing in the morning or right before bedtime. Drink plenty of water.

COENZYME Q10
Background information: Japanese studies have found that coenzyme Q10 supplementation stimulates the production of insulin and glucose utilization.

Typical dosage: 50 to 80 mg daily.

MANGANESE

Background information: A deficiency of manganese can lead to glucose intolerance but can be reversed through supplementation. The levels of manganese in diabetics are half those in normal people.

Typical dosage: 5 to 10 mg daily.

GYMNEMA SYLVESTRE

Background information: This herb has an extensive history as a traditional treatment for obesity and blood sugar disorders. Known as the "destroyer of sugar," it contains gymnemic acid, which has the unique ability to inhibit the taste of sugar. Because its chemical structure is so similar to glucose, it actually binds with sugar receptors contained in our mouths. After eating this herb, sweet foods become virtually tasteless and lose their appeal.

Typical dosage: If using gymnema to inhibit the taste of sweet foods, use a tea or liquid extract form of the herb. Remember that gymnema's effect will only last for a maximum of two hours, so it should be taken fifteen minutes prior to eating so that sweet foods will lose their appeal. If you do not want your taste buds to be desensitized to sweet foods but want the insulin-enhancing benefits of the herb, take 400 mg of gymnema daily, 200 mg at breakfast and 200 mg at lunch. Look for standardized herbal supplements that contain 24 percent gymnemic acid in capsule form.

Also remember that regular exercise helps to normalize insulin resistance and works to prevent conditions like Type II diabetes, which is directly linked to obesity.

CHAPTER 8

Food Allergies and Mood Disorders

One man's meat is another man's poison.
LUCRETIUS, FIRST CENTURY B.C. POET

THE PREVIOUS CHAPTER provided some compelling evidence that the relationship between food and behavior is a real one. Moreover, the effects of food on behavior vary from person to person. In other words, what can be eaten by one person without any side effects, can cause another person to feel and act lousy. In fact, several prominent physicians have linked food allergies to depression—not to mention migraines, schizophrenia, arthritis, obesity and eczema. Conventional medicine, on the other hand, refutes the connection. Like hypoglycemia, the existence of food allergies is still questioned by some physicians, and the entire notion that food sensitivities cause behavioral or mood disorders has received a cool reception within the scientific community.

Michel de Montaigne explains it well:

> Whenever a new discovery is reported to the scientific world, they say first, "It is probably not true." Thereafter, when the truth of the new proposition has been demonstrated beyond question, they say, "Yes, it may be true, but it is not important." Finally, when sufficient time has elapsed to fully evidence its importance they say, "Yes, surely it is important, but it is no longer new."

Accepted or not, however, food sensitivities do exist and seem to be on the rise. No doubt, factors such as breathing polluted air, ingesting hidden chemical and toxic metals in food and water, undergoing stress, and having poor dietary habits have contributed to the development of these hypersensitivities.

Nevertheless, physicians rarely acknowledge food allergies as a health problem, let alone pursue the possibility that a food allergy may be causing your melancholy. Harvey Ross, M.D., puts it this way:

> One major flaw of modern psychiatry is the exclusive pursuit of psychotherapy or drug therapy for patients who lack energy and clear thinking. Such problems often have nutritional causes, and when treated, facilitate psychotherapy tremendously or even eliminate the need for it . . . to unravel problems effectively, it is necessary to explore how and what a person eats, not just his family history and potentially significant emotional events.

In fact, you will probably discover that a large part of puzzle-solving depression is diet. Analyzing what goes into your body and how what you eat affects your body (and your mind) is essential to recovery. It takes time to put together all the pieces, but it is the best way to attack depression at its source.

It is important to remember before beginning that effective treatment of any food sensitivity depends on the total elimination of the targeted food. If you eliminate suspect foods, you should feel better within a few weeks. Dr. Ross believes that after abstaining from these foods for several months, they may be slowly re-introduced into the diet as long as they are only eaten occasionally.

How Do You Define a Food Allergy?

Simply stated, a food allergy is intolerance to a certain food or foods. This kind of allergy does not bring on the same symptoms we normally associate with allergies—watery, itchy eyes, sneezing, wheezing, hives, and runny nose. For this reason, food allergies are difficult to pinpoint. Because symptoms vary from person to person and reactions are often delayed, food allergies may not be identified for what they really are. Although it's easy to identify food sensitivities with symptoms like hives, mouth sores, or asthma, linking food to emotional states is much more difficult.

Many nutritionists now openly accept the fact that food allergies frequently cause hyperkinetic behavior in children. In these instances, children with attention deficit hyperactivity disorder (ADHD) are immediately taken off of sugar, wheat and dairy products because there is substantial evidence that hyperactivity is related to what one eats. In other words, certain kinds of food can wreak havoc in a sensitive person's brain chemistry. Elisa Lotter, Ph.D., relates the story of Henry, who at age seventeen had been treated with tranquilizers, electric shock treatments and psychotherapy for several years with no significant improvement. He was subsequently placed on a strict fast and was given only spring water. After four days, he experienced a complete reversal of symptoms, until the fifth day, when he was given a meal consisting of wheat only. Within an hour, he began to experience negative, paranoid thoughts. Further testing confirmed that when certain foods were withheld from Henry, his symptoms disappeared and when they were added, he became mentally disturbed again.

Likewise, Drs. Philpott and Kalita, in their book *Brain Allergies,* discuss the very significant mental impact that dairy products and cereal grains have on some schizophrenics. The implication here is that hidden food sensitivities may be responsible for a number of emotional disorders in susceptible people. The very nature of what we eat is often unknown to us. In other words, we very willingly open microwaveable dinners or brightly colored boxes and bags and eagerly consume a number of mystery ingredients and chemicals. Marshall Mandell, M.D., who has written two books and numerous scientific papers on the subject of food intolerances, says that when natural food substances are tampered with, they can become contaminants rather than nutrients to the body. He states, "Furthermore, contemporary mass-production strips food of many valuable nutrients that, were they left intact, would provide protective benefits."

Apparently, there are several ways a food allergy can trigger a mood change. During an allergic reaction, the body leaks histamine from the capillaries, which can cause edema or swelling around them. This phenomenon is understood by those who suffer from pollen allergies. If you have hay fever, your sinuses swell and you can't breathe through your nose. Dr. Mandell believes that the same reaction can take place in brain cells when you eat a culprit food, causing a disruption in brain chemistry. In the same way that muscle spasms cause the bronchiole tubes to constrict during an allergic asthma attack, he proposes that similar spasms in the small arteries of the brain can reduce the flow of glucose, oxygen and other nutrients to brain tissue. Both of these scenarios would naturally cause a change in behavior or mood.

If you have allergies to certain foods, you won't experience just a change in mood. In fact, like the role of sugar in hypoglycemia, you may initially be stimulated by eating a food you are allergic to. Symptoms are frequently delayed and therefore, often misdiagnosed.

Symptoms of Food Sensitivities

Billy Casper, famous for his golfing, complained for years of weight gain, gastric aliments, sinus congestion, backaches, headaches and a bad temper. Apparently, after some investigation and testing, he was found to be sensitive to beet sugar, lamb, apples, pork, eggs, citrus fruit, wheat and any fruits or vegetables fertilized with nitrates or sprayed with chemicals. When Billy made significant alterations to his lifestyle and his diet, his health—particularly his moods—significantly improved.

Like Billy Casper, for many adults the most common symptoms of a food allergy are depression, headaches and fatigue. Mood changes can range from mild forms of anxiety to serious depression. Manic outbursts of uncontrollable anger are also a possible symptom of food intolerance. As mentioned earlier, the relationship between food allergies and schizophrenia is currently under investigation.

Mold: The Hidden Culprit

Mold is one example of a disguised food intolerance. For instance, it may not be cheese that you are allergic to, but rather the mold that grows on it. Mold-containing foods may cause a variety of symptoms from headache to fatigue. Keeping food properly stored can help decrease mold growth. Foods that can contain mold include buttermilk, beer, canned tomato products, cheeses, dehydrated fruits, mushrooms, sourdough and rye breads, and products that contain vinegar, wine and yogurt.

If you eat a food that you are sensitive to, one of two reactions will occur. An immediate effect is characterized by easily recognizable symptoms that develop shortly after consumption. For instance, if you eat shrimp and break out in hives or develop an unusual headache, you know the shrimp is probably responsible. However, the second type of food reaction is more difficult to identify because it may not occur for a day or two. For example, if you ate a large meal on Sunday, you may feel fatigued, lethargic and depressed on Tuesday. In these cases, connecting your symptoms with a meal you ate a couple of days ago is unlikely. Several medical journals in the 1980s published articles which proposed that delayed food allergies caused a significant number of migraine headaches. In addition, reports in the *Journal of Arthritis and Rheumatism* disclosed that many cases of rheumatoid and osteoarthritis cleared up when certain offending foods were removed from the diet.

Food Allergies Impact Behavior

Numerous studies connect allergic reactions to mood. Abram Hoffer, M.D., reported in an article published in the *Journal of Orthomolecular Psychiatry* that "treatment of the allergy will, in

The Autism Connection to Sugar Malabsorption

Just to emphasize the importance of proper digestion and assimilation of food, a 1999 issue of the *Journal of Pediatrics* reported that gastrointestinal malfunctions have been linked to autism in some children. Researchers at the University of Maryland concluded that unrecognized gastrointestinal disorders, especially the malabsorption of certain sugars, may contribute to the behavioral problems of some autistic children who can't communicate verbally. They recommended further research be done to determine the link between the brain and the digestive system and to shed more light on this surprising connection.

most cases, cure the depression. I have seen this in several hundred patients." Although the exact way an allergic reaction to food changes brain function is still a mystery, the link between the two still exists in research.

Explanations have surfaced to explain this link, and include the idea of swollen brain cells and serotonin changes. Another theory is explained by Michael B. Schachter, M.D., in his book *Food, Mind and Mood*. He suggests that in certain people, specific foods may stimulate the body's production of antibodies, which can clump together and collect in the blood vessels of the brain. As a result, brain cells become oxygen deprived, causing a variety of mood and behavioral changes. Scandinavian scientists published a 1997 study that supports this theory. Scientists reported that when food-sensitive individuals eat certain foods, the immune system kicks in and stimulates physical and behavioral reactions. Their double-blind study found that people with food sensitivities are at higher risk for depression, anxiety, shyness and defensiveness.

Austrian researchers recently offered another theory. They recently published their work reporting that people who do not absorb fructose (fruit sugar) properly can become clinically depressed. When these people eat fruit, its fructose content is broken down in the colon by bacteria into short fatty acids, CO_2 and H_2. Bloating, cramps, diarrhea and other symptoms of irritable bowel syndrome usually occurred, as well as increased PMS and depression. They concluded that fructose malabsorption may play a role in the development of depressed mood and should be addressed by doctors who see depressed patients.

While there is still much work to do in this field, I cannot help but believe that some foods trigger a domino effect in sensitive individuals that impacts brain chemistry, mood and behavior. For instance, celiac disease is caused by a food intolerance to any grain that contains gluten or gluten-like substances. The disease progressively causes the destruction of the surface of the small bowel, where nutrients are absorbed. Any time a person with this disease eats a food they can't tolerate, more colon cell destruction occurs. Depression is common to people suffering from celiac disease, and various studies have linked this depression with a lack of vitamin B6. They have found that treating the depression with vitamin B6 supplements can be quite successful.

Food Allergies Can Be Easily Misdiagnosed

Because the symptoms are so similar, it is easy to mistake a food allergy for hypoglycemia. Both are directly related to an improper diet and share the same type of relationship with meals. In addition, a food allergy can cause an abnormal insulin response, which could show up as hypoglycemia on a glucose tolerance test. Also, both hypoglycemia and food allergies can often be controlled by restricting highly refined carbohydrates and grains like wheat.

Dr. Mandell's study of 200 hospitalized schizophrenics found that 65 percent were sensitive to wheat products, and 50 percent to milk and corn products. He also found that the most frequently craved and eaten foods continually resulted in the worst symptoms. In addition, the amount of a food and how often it was eaten played a significant role. In other words, a certain food eaten once a week may be tolerated by the body; however, if it is eaten every day, it may cause symptoms to develop.

How Do You Become Food Intolerant?

How does one develop a food allergy? You can actually become sensitive to the foods that you have spent years overeating. The theory is that eventually this particular food becomes dangerous to the body because it is perceived as an allergen, just like pollen. Even more interesting is the research done on food allergies.

Research has determined that frequently the body craves the very food that causes it to feel ill. If you stop eating a certain food you have consumed for years, you can develop a set of symptoms that are not relieved until you eat that particular food again. Talk about a vicious cycle!

Foods that are commonly associated with allergic reactions include cow's milk products, wheat, eggs, yeast, corn, soy, cane sugar, dyes and preservatives. It is not uncommon to also become allergic to beef, chicken, lettuce, artificial sweeteners and tobacco. There has been some speculation that even the water we consume may cause allergic reactions in some people. For this reason, if you find that you are food sensitive, use bottled water rather than chlorinated or fluoridated supplies.

A List of Foods Commonly Associated with Allergic Reactions

When assessing food sensitivities and depression, it is important to note that gluten is at the top of the intolerance list. A gluten intolerance, even a mild one, has been cited as a plausible cause of depression. Dr. Alan Gaby, M.D., states that gluten intolerance—a sensitivity to wheat, oats, barley and rye—may be much more common than previously assumed. The following are some of the most common culprits involved in food allergies.

• berry fruits or fruit peelings
• chocolate
• corn and corn by-products (i.e. corn syrup, sweeteners, oil)
• dairy products

• eggs
• food additives and preservatives (especially MSG)
• nuts
• shellfish
• wheat products
• yeast

Food Additives Recognized as Safe by the FDA

Most of us would agree that as a nation, we eat an enormous amount of processed and preserved foods. In fact, what we refer to as "food" sometimes is a real stretch of the imagination. Michael Jacobson in the April 1975 edition of *Smithsonian* stated:

> The United States, not surprisingly, has been the leader in the genetic engineering of food crops and in the laboratory creation of new foods. Benjamin Franklin and Abraham Lincoln, if they could visit us, would probably have some difficulty distinguishing between a toy store and a supermarket. They would not even recognize products like artificial whipped cream in its pressurized can, or some breakfast "cereals" that are almost half sugar and bear little resemblance to cereal grains . . . Many of the new foods do save us time and trouble, but they are often costly, in terms of both dollars and, ultimately, health.

Needless to say, there are countless chemicals added to our foods, and determining which chemicals are causing reactions in your body can be difficult. Table 1 lists a few of the thousands of additives currently recognized as safe by the FDA. You may find that eliminating as many additives as possible is more effective than trying to narrow down a particular offending additive.

A NOTE ON MSG

There's a good reason many of us feel wasted after eating Chinese food. MSG is a flavor enhancer commonly used in Chinese food that can cause symptoms from a simple headache and numbness to sudden depression, heart palpitations and

Table 1. Sampling of food additives recognized
as safe by the FDA.

Acacia gum	Diacetyl	Magnesium
Acetic acid	Diethyl succinate	Chloride
Acetone	Ethyl acetate	MSG
Allyl disulfide	Ethyl cellulose	Myristic acid
Aluminum sulfate	Fatty acids	Nitrogen
Ammonium chlo-	Fatty alcohols,	Olestra (Olean)
ride	synthetic	Paraffin wax
Anisyl alcohol	Ferric chloride	Peptones
Aspartame	Gelatin	Petroleum wax
Bentonite	Geraniol	Potassium bromate
Benzoyl peroxide	Glycerin	Propyl alcohol
Bromelain	Ground limestone	Quinine sulfate
Brominated veg-	Haw bark extract	Rubber, natural-
etable oil	Heptylparaben	smoked sheet
Butter acids	High-fructose corn	Saccharin
Butyl alcohol	syrup	Salicylaldehyde
Caffeine	Hydrochloric acid	Sodium benzoate
Calcium peroxide	Hydrogenated veg-	Sodium nitrite
Camphene	etable oil	Sorbitol
Carbon dioxide	5-Hydroxy-4-	Starch
Carmine	Octanone	Sucralose
Carnauba wax	Invert sugar	Sulfuric acid
Casein	Ion exchange resin	Titanium dioxide
Castor oil	Iron ammonium	Terpentine, steam
Cetyl alcohol	citrate	instilled
Chlorine dioxide	Isobutyl alcohol	Urea
Citronella oil	Lactic acid	Xanthophyll
Clay, attapulgite	Lactose	Xylenol
Copper sulfate	Lanolin	Zinc sulfate
Dextrose	L-Limonene	

From: EAFUS(Everything Added to Food in the United States), a food additive database maintained by the FDA's Center for Food Safety and Applied Nutrition (CFSAN) under a program known as Priority-based Assessment of Food Additives (PAFA) severe weakness. MSG is a chemical form of glutamic acid, an amino acid used as a building block of protein. When susceptible people get inordinate amounts of MSG, they can experience negative bodily reactions. Personally speaking, if I eat food with MSG, I become anxious and irritable. To be on the safe side, avoid this food additive.

What to Do if You Suspect a Food Allergy

Typically, when we keep eating foods that our body is sensitive to, we create a vicious cycle of symptoms that we can't trace to one source or time. For this reason, going on an elimination diet is probably the most effective way to pinpoint the foods that cause you to feel lousy, and it is an excellent example of how to apply the puzzle-solving process. The premise of the diet is simple: when you stop eating certain foods, you will feel markedly better.

Begin by compiling a list of suspicious foods, especially foods that you eat a lot. Generally speaking, each food you eliminate should not be eaten for at least a week to make sure that no trace of than food remains in the body. Eliminating foods for two to six weeks is even better. Also, test only one food at a time. While this is far from an exact science, it should give you a better idea of which foods could be problematic. By systematically removing a food and then reintroducing it, you should be able to tell if a particular food (or set of foods) is causing the problem.

What is challenging about this type of test is uncovering hidden ingredients in foods that may be causing the trouble. As mentioned earlier, mold on certain foods or food additives could be a problem. Drugs, supplements or even tap water may also contribute to allergic reactions and must be taken into consideration. After doing basic testing on your favorite foods, however, you can also test other, more hidden, aspects of your diet.

Sometimes only one or two foods need to be excluded, and certain foods have a track record for causing specific disorders. For example, a sensitivity to gluten—found in rye, barley, oats and wheat—has been linked to celiac disease. Because of this, it is also important to keep in mind that when you begin an elimination diet, you will most likely go through an adjustment period when symptoms actually get worse. This usually happens within a day of beginning the program. Some people feel downright sick. What this suggests is that the foods excluded are indeed problem foods. In time, if you don't break down and eat them again, you will start to feel better.

After a few weeks or a month, you can begin to reintroduce single foods and watch your symptoms. Don't reintroduce foods too quickly, and keep a journal of what you eat, when you eat it, and how you feel afterwards. Try to find patterns or consistencies with certain foods and subsequent symptoms over time.

If you don't have the time or patience for an elimination diet, blood tests to determine food sensitivities are also available. They are designed to detect cellular changes or immune responses to certain foods, but although they are convenient, they can be costly and are not totally reliable. At best, they can give you a place to start by suggesting the most likely foods that cause trouble. Skin scratch tests are also available; however, they are only limited to skin reactions that are rarely involved in food sensitivities. Skin testing for food allergies is highly ineffective, and the reliability of pendulum swings and electro-acupuncture are still questionable.

In certain parts of the country, a blood test is available that measures the presence of the immunoglobulin G (IgG) and may also help to determine if you have a food allergy. This test is called the IgE-IgG RAST test or the ELISA/ACT test. The availability of the cytotoxic test has also made it possible to investigate and discover food sensitivities with greater accuracy and ease. This particular test must be performed by a qualified technician, however. Also, bear in mind that the test is never 100 percent accurate.

Perhaps one of the easiest ways to determine if you are suffering from a food allergy is to keep track of your pulse rate after eating. Sit quietly and count the number of beats that occur in a minute. A normal pulse is between fifty to seventy beats per minute. After you have recorded your pulse, eat the food in question. Wait twenty minutes and take your pulse again. If you find that you pulse rate has increased within ten beats, omit this food from your diet, and then try this food and the test again later. Also, try to keep the foods that you test as simple as possible and in their purest and most simple form.

You can also purchase special testing strips that can help determine the presence of sulfites. Ask you pharmacist about this home test kit. For more information on test strips to detect the presence of sulfites in foods write to: Sulfitest, Center Laboratories, 35 Channel Drive, Port Washington, NY 11050 or call (800) 645-6335.

Whichever method you choose, I recommend keeping a food journal where you can list everything you eat and how you felt afterwards. (And remember, that what you ate on the weekend can determine how you feel on Monday morning.) Keeping a record like a food diary enables you to eliminate individual foods for certain time periods and assess your symptoms, as well as determining if certain groups of food eaten together cause the symptoms. Although it can be somewhat time consuming, it is an excellent way to pinpoint culprit foods. And the problem-solving techniques you learn from careful analysis of your diet will help you as you piece together other factors contributing to your depression.

Supplement Game Plan for Treating Food Intolerance (Use with Core Protocol)

VITAMIN C WITH QUERCETIN (A BIOFLAVONOID)
Note: This can replace the vitamin C recommendation listed in the Core Protocol.
Typical dosage: (Vitamin C) 10,000 to 20,000 mg per day divided into two or more doses. Ascorbic acid can be purchased in powdered form for larger than normal dosages. People who suffer from allergies can often tolerate megadoses of vitamin C. If stomach upset is a problem, use buffered forms of vitamin C. (Quercetin) 1 to 2 grams daily divided into three to six doses.

HISTIDINE
Typical dosage: 200 mg once daily

VITAMIN B5 (PANTOTHENIC ACID)
Typical dosage: 500 mg with meals

MSM (METHYL SULFONYL METHANE)
Typical dosage: 250 to 500 mg per day. Because MSM initiates cellular cleansing, you may feel worse initially, but with continued supplementation, you should see improvement.

CHAPTER 9

The Colon Connection to Depression

Many degenerative diseases are brought about by toxins generated in the large bowel. Bacterial flora imbalance, putrefaction of undigested foods, parasitic and yeast infections may be at the bottom (excuse the pun) of many diseases.

ZOLTON P. RONA, M.D., M.SC.

RECENTLY, A STUDY from the Department of Pediatrics at the University of Massachusetts reported that constipation may cause children to misbehave. Researchers observed that in the group of children whose constipation was treated, there were improvements in the children's self-esteem, moods, anxiety and irritability levels. While it seems unlikely that what goes on down in your intestines can impact your mental attitude—be assured that it can. If the data cited in this book has done nothing else, it should at least demonstrate the complex and fragile interconnection that exists among all of our body systems. In other words, no organ is an island.

The health of your colon is determined in part by what you put in your mouth. For instance, did you know that what you eat determines the kind of bacteria found in your intestines? If you eat a lot of complex carbohydrates and very little protein, your intestinal flora will primarily consists of bacteria that breakdown carbohydrates. On the other hand, if your diet is high in protein and low in carbohydrates, intestinal bacteria will be of the proteolytic type, which is designed to decompose proteins. In fact, some scientists believe that proteolytic bacteria can transform the amino acids that come from protein foods we eat into powerful toxins. If we were regularly and thoroughly moving waste out of the bowel, the risk for putrefaction and toxin build-up would be less. Realistically speaking, however, most of us suffer from chronic constipation. Consequently, a condition called intestinal toxemia can develop. Consider the fact that if you eat ninety-four grams of protein per day (the amount eaten by a large number of Americans), this digested protein waste can remain in the large intestines for a long time. And because most of us eat low-fiber diets, we only compound the problem. As a result, adverse chemical reactions can occur in the colon. Eating a lot of meat, in particular, can create delayed elimination, which in turn causes a number of poisons to form in the colon. The colon then adversely affects other body systems, including the brain.

High-Protein Diets Create Colon Toxicity

When you eat a diet rich in meat, the amino acid tyrosine is converted to phenol, and the tryptophan is converted to indole and skatole in the bowel. Remember that tyrosine and tryptophan are precursor compounds to the brain chemicals that control mood. These by-products are considered toxic and are believed to re-enter the bloodstream to some extent. When this happens, the liver tries to detoxify them, but phenol can elude this filtering process and may continue to circulate in the bloodstream.

It is the presence of phenol that some experts believe is responsible for a whole host of ailments, including allergies, autoimmune diseases like arthritis and lupus, cancer, back pain and mental illness. This intestinal phenomenon is referred to as autointoxication and is gaining more credibility among medical doctors.

Furthermore, mainstream medicine has finally accepted the notion that eating too much protein is bad for human beings—a fact that was taught in the early twentieth century to doctors by respected medical colleagues. A paper read at the annual meeting of the American Medical Association in 1917 reported 517 cases of mental symptoms that were relieved by eliminating intestinal toxemia. Some of these mental symptoms that were listed at the 1917 medical convention were nervousness, fatigue and "general wretchedness," a particularly good way to describe depression itself. Then, in 1962, experts looked at these toxic bowel chemicals and linked them to schizophrenia.

In fact, we now know that a high-protein diet aggravates colon disease. Eating a diet rich in complex carbohydrates (raw fruits, vegetables and whole grains) and lower in protein is accepted as an overall healthier way to eat. Eating this way results in a decrease of proteolytic bacteria responsible for autointoxication. To put it simply, we were not designed to dine on steak every night.

We should be eating fifty grams of protein per day rather than the typical ninety-four, and some health care experts recommend eating as few as 25 or 30 grams per day if you're not a child, pregnant, or nursing. However, I believe if you eat soy foods, this amount is too low. It is the overconsumption of meat that is linked to colon disorders. Soy foods actually contain some of the healthiest forms of protein you can consume.

What Constitutes Constipation?

Although significant controversy still exists over how often a healthy colon should eliminate waste, it is generally accepted that bowel movements should occur every twelve to eighteen hours. For years, we've associated a grumpy disposition with constipation. Few of us knew, however, that prolonged constipation may be a contributing factor to depressed mental states.

We take more laxatives in this country than anywhere else in the world. This fact alone should be a wake-up call. It illustrates that more often than not, what we choose to eat taxes our bodies rather than sustains them. Constipation is not a normal condition. Being continually constipated can significantly taint the way we view life and its challenges, not to mention drain our energy reserves. Many

> ## Antibiotic Overkill?
>
> New data reveals that millions of Americans routinely overuse antibiotics for everything from a cold to a hangnail. This glut of flora-killing drugs is setting us up for a frightening array of disease-resistant bacteria. Antibiotics can save lives, but that doesn't change the fact that they are grossly overprescribed. In fact, some antibiotics are actually linked to depression, and their use can create chaos with the digestive tract. Anyone taking a course of antibiotics should also take acidophilus in the form of active-culture yogurt or supplementation to replace lost intestinal bacteria. Without it, we become susceptible to infection, poor digestion and constipation.

people who are constipated also suffer from colon disorders like irritable bowel syndrome.

Colon Disease and Depression

How exactly is the colon linked with depression? Evidence suggests that people who suffer from bowel disorders—like chronic constipation or diarrhea, irritable bowel syndrome, spastic colon or colitis—may also be victims of vitamin B6 deficiencies. When the bowel is irritated or sluggish, the effectiveness of nutrient absorption is also impaired to some extent. Over an extended period of time, this impairment can cause deficiencies in the body. As previously established, poor B-vitamin absorption can affect mental outlook. In fact, a study published in a 1999 issue of *Psychosomatic Medicine* reported that psychiatric illness is higher among people with irritable bowel syndrome. The researchers concluded that female patients in particular had a high incidence of clinical depression associated with irritable bowel syndrome.

Another new study published in a 1999 issue of the *Journal of Gastroenterology* has found similar link between fibromyalgia and irritable bowel syndrome. Fibromyalgia is another mystery disease that mostly affects women and is closely associated with depression. The irritable bowel component of this disease may shed new light on why mood slumps are so common in women suffering from fibromyalgia.

Irritable bowel syndrome and other colon-related ailments are extremely common in the United States, and perhaps the epidemic proportions of depression experienced in this country are due, to some extent, to the high prevalence of colon disease. The typical American diet is high in animal fat, dairy products and refined carbohydrates, which perpetuate colon disorders.

Supplement Game Plan for Treating Digestive Disorders (Use with Core Protocol)

FIBER
Typical dosage: 30 grams of fiber daily from sources like bran, fiber supplement drinks and fresh fruits and vegetables (i.e. apples, raspberries, artichokes)

CASCARA SAGRADA (RHAMNUS PURSHIANA)
Typical dosage: Take as directed. Use a supplement from a reputable distributor since the bark must be aged correctly to be effective. This herb is derived from a tree bark that increases the peristalsis of the colon and has been used for generations to treat constipation. Cascara sagrada is considered one of the most effective herbal treatments of chronic constipation because it is not habit forming. In addition, this herb is believed to function as a tonic for the nerves and contains B vitamins, calcium, potassium and manganese.

MAGNESIUM (BOUND TO CITRATE, MALATE, FUMARATE, SUCCINATE OR ASPARTATE)
Typical dosage: 250 mg three times daily

PRUNE JUICE
Typical dosage: 8 ounces daily

ACIDOPHILUS
Typical dosage: Take as directed using milk-free, guaranteed bacterial count products with bifidobacteria. Check for expiration date, and take on an empty stomach. This supplement replenishes friendly bacteria in the bowel and controls gas and bloating. Studies have found that it can relieve symptoms associated with colitis and irritable bowel syndrome

DIGESTIVE OR PROTEOLYTIC ENZYMES (PANCREATIN, PEPSIN AND BROMELAIN)
Typical dosage: Take as directed on an empty stomach thirty minutes before meals and before going to bed. Enteric-coated bromelain and other enzymes may be preferable for bowel treatment. These compounds help you more thoroughly digest food and avoid the retention of undigested protein particles that can initiate food allergies and cause constipation or diarrhea.

GINGER ROOT
Typical dosage: Use 5 to 10 grams of fresh ginger root daily or take 200 mg of a ginger supplement standardized to a 20 percent gingerol content three times daily. Ginger oil can also be used to enhance massage therapy. Ginger is one of the best herbs for the treatment of digestive disorders. Ginger prevents nausea, gas, bloating and intestinal cramping.

WATER
Typical dosage: Drink at least six eight-ounce glasses of pure water daily.

CHAPTER 10

The Female Face of Depression

TWICE AS MANY women as men get depressed. Postpartum and postmenopausal women, as well as women on the pill, are prime candidates for depression. Research tell us that women internalize their problems more than men. A recent study conducted at the Department of Psychology at the University of Michigan in Ann Arbor found that women more than men, feel that they have lost control of their lives. Women also have a tendency to "ruminate" or dwell on their problems more than men. This study appeared in a 1999 issue of the *Journal of Personality and Social Psychology* and looked at 1,100 men and women from twenty-five to seventy-five years old in three California cities over a period of two years. In the end, it was concluded that women who had the highest levels of stress and rumination also had the highest levels of depression.

In addition, if a woman has less decision-making ability or money, the situation is even worse. Combine that scenario with the hormonal roller coaster women often experience, and you have all the ingredients needed for serious depression. In fact, approximately one in four women will experience some type of depression during their lives. While some experts believe these statistics are not accurate—women may just admit to being depressed more often than men, my experience supports the available data. And depressive illness affects women regardless of their racial, cultural or economic background, and this holds true in several countries.

I believe that the main reason for this difference is the monthly hormonal flux women experience, which obviously impacts their brain chemistry. Pregnancy and delivery affect neurotransmitter production in the brain. In fact, studies reported in the *British Medical Journal* show that women who suffer from post-menopausal depression and younger women who suffer from PMS depression prior to their periods have impaired tryptophan metabolism, which is linked to the production of serotonin and positive moods.

If you are a depressed female, hormones could be an instrumental piece to your depression. This chapter will help you investigate the effect of hormone imbalance on mood, and it will offer you solutions to various factors that can affect mood. Of course, identifying your triggers and experimenting with solutions can take time, but if there is even a chance that your depression is connected to hormones, it is important to invest the time in addressing potential problems.

Girls Tend to Become Depressed Early

For many women, depression begins during adolescence when peer pressure and expectations color notions of female self-value, identity and sexuality. It is generally thought that girls are more dramatically impacted by these issues than adolescent boys, though that sentiment is changing. Nevertheless, adolescent girls and boys do seem to internalize teenage experiences differently, which could explain their often differing reactions to these life events.

The traits that contribute to the likelihood of getting depressed include pessimism, low self-esteem, excessive worrying and feelings of helplessness. For a variety of reasons, girls seem more prone to experience these emotions, and they can develop depressed thought patterns early that can predispose them to a lifetime battle with depression.

As young women mature, many continue to struggle with issues that arose during adolescence, such as weight, beauty and success, as well as job performance, mothering, marriage and other everyday demands that can create an enormous amount of physical and emotional stress. Women also have a tendency to assess their self-worth based on the success of their relationships with others. All of these factors coupled with monthly hormonal swings or menopausal issues can create a prime environment for depression.

Factors that Make Women More Vulnerable to Depression

The rest of this section will address the different factors that can influence mood in women. At the end of the chapter are a number of treatments for problems related to hormonal imbalance. Apply your puzzle-solving skills carefully as you read through the following pages. One or a number of these pieces could cause depression.

Stress and Cortisol

Some experts claim that up to 90 percent of all illnesses are stress related. Depression is no exception. Because women have a tendency to expect so much from themselves, their stress levels often skyrocket—setting them up for depressive illness. Many women find themselves juggling homemaking, parenting, a job, and caring for aged parents all in the course of one day, and many of these same women fail to eat nutritiously. Some of these women may try to exercise to keep their weight down, but they do so without adequate nutritional support. In addition, women who are overworked or who deal with significant worries often fail to sleep soundly at night. Poor sleep compounds the problems of depression. All of these factors leave the average woman less able to handle their daily stresses.

When we are stressed, more of a hormone called cortisol is secreted from the adrenal glands. Cortisol contributes to protein building and regulates insulin, among other things. Under conditions of stress, however, high amounts of cortisol are released. These high cortisol levels have been linked to weight gain, low thyroid function, muscle and joint pain, and depression.

The CRH (corticotropin-releasing hormone) controls how much cortisol is produced by the body at various sites, including the brain. Scientists have found that under periods of stress, this hormone stays elevated continually, which can adversely effect both the mind and the body, leading to both anxiety and depression.

Learning to diffuse stress, then, is very important for all women. Using meditation, massage and exercise on a regular basis helps to negate the dangerous effects of stress. I believe that female stress has escalated to a crisis point and certainly accounts for a woman's tendency to become depressed. Moreover, if you endured prolonged periods of stress as a child, your brain functions can become altered, causing future behavioral and/or mood problems.

The Impact of Abuse on Women

Women who were sexually abused as children are more likely to have clinical depression at some time in their lives compared to those who were not. According to the American Psychological Association's Task Force on Women and Depression, 37 percent of depressed women had suffered significant physical or sexual abuse by age twenty-one.

In addition, women who were raped also showed a much higher tendency toward depression. Guilt, self-degradation and isolation can all contribute to these women's mood disorders and need to be addressed by qualified counselors.

Moreover, the role of suppressed rage or anger must also be considered as an underlying theme in some cases of depression. Some of us deal with feelings of overwhelming anger by becoming passive and unresponsive, by withdrawing and slipping down into a place where that rage won't manifest itself. Our brains don't know what to do with all that anger and resentment, and so consciously or not, we retreat to a place where we can feel no emotion. If you believe your depression may stem from abuse, see a counselor and get some professional help. Be aware that your depression is not just an emotional by-product of past trauma. Abuse can change the landscape of the brain.

ABUSE ALTERS THE CHEMICAL STRUCTURE OF THE BRAIN

To further illustrate just how damaging abuse can be, consider the fact that when someone physically or verbally abuses us—or if we witness abuse between our parents or other family members, the chemical topography of our brain changes. For anyone who struggles with an abusive past, this fact is very important to realize. Your current depression may well have its roots in changes your brain experienced as a child.

Prolonged stress can have the same effect. For example, some new studies suggest that the alarming incidence of ADHD in American children could be the result of impaired brain chemistry due to certain stressors. One recent study found that compounds that release cortisol (the stress hormone) from the adrenal glands may manipulate areas of the brain that determine how we behave when we feel stressed. Any malfunction of this system may be the key to understanding conditions such as drug or alcohol abuse, eating disorders, anxiety attacks of depression—all of which are considered abnormal reactions to stress.

Hormonal Flux and Mood

In addition to daily stress, the ebb and tide of a woman's hormonal landscape inevitably impacts her mental state. The menstrual cycle, pregnancy, postpartum, infertility issues and menopause can all contribute to periods of depression. We now know that reproductive hormones have a profound effect on the brain chemistry and how a woman feels emotionally.

Naturally, when we think of mood disorders associated with hormones, PMS comes to mind. Some women experience very low moods during this time interval, although the exact mechanism involved is not totally understood.

Baby blues can also initiate serious depressive illness. Some woman can slip into a depression deep enough to completely incapacitate them. Remember that the dramatic hormonal transition that occurs after childbirth coupled with possible nutrient deficiencies such as a lack of folic acid or vitamin B6 can make the problem even worse.

Women facing menopause can also be prone to mood disorders, although some experts believe that only women who have had a prior history of depression will face menopausal melancholia. Many theories have been proposed to explain this fact, but it's obvious to me that circulating levels of estrogen and progesterone have a profound impact on brain chemistry and mood. Working to maintain hormonal balance, in combination with nutritious eating, can go a long way to stave off hormonally induced depression. I believe one of the most common hormonal problems premenopausal (and sometimes menopausal) women face is estrogen dominance.

Estrogen Dominance

When estrogen is unopposed or unbalanced by progesterone, the results can be undesirable, annoying, and even dangerous. Progesterone is the hormone that helps modulate the negative effects of estrogen. Keep in mind that even a low amount of estrogen will dominate if it is not properly balanced with adequate levels of progesterone.

If you find that you continually battle cyclic depression, anger or deep-seated resentment, you may suffer from PMS—a condition that is directly related to estrogen overload. Look over the following lists of both physical and emotional signs of estrogen dominance to see if you fit the profile.

PHYSICAL SYMPTOMS OF ESTROGEN DOMINANCE

- breast enlargement and tenderness
- carbohydrate cravings
- certain types of acne
- cold hands and feet
- fibrocystic breasts
- fibroid tumors
- headaches
- heavy menstrual flow or irregular periods
- hypoglycemia
- inability to maintain a pregnancy
- infertility
- thyroid dysfunction
- uterine cramping
- uterine fibroids
- water retention
- weight gain (fat on hips and thighs)

EMOTIONAL SYMPTOMS OF ESTROGEN DOMINANCE

- depression
- fatigue
- inability to focus
- loss of libido
- mood swings
- quick to anger

ESTROGEN, MOOD AND SEROTONIN

The delicate relationship between amino acids, vitamins and neurotransmitters discussed earlier in this book is further complicated by the presence of estrogen. As you can see from the list above, an estrogen overload can cause a number of distressing symptoms, including depression. Estrogen is a central nervous stimulant while progesterone has the opposite effect. Maintaining the right balance between these two hormones is a complex and delicate process.

Estrogen's Effect on Serotonin Production

The tryptophan link to serotonin is also influenced by estrogen. In order to have enough serotonin, you need to consume adequate amounts of tryptophan (an amino acid). To maintain optimal levels of tryptophan in the body, it must be supplied with certain amounts of vitamin B6. Estrogen can block the action of vitamin B6 and force it to be eliminated from the body. It can also speed up the production of tryptophan, which, ironically, makes it less likely to convert to serotonin.

Interestingly, too little estrogen can also wreak emotional havoc. A study recently published in a 1999 issue of *Psychopharmacology* reported that when estradiol (a form of estrogen) dips, it causes the type of depression commonly seen in postpartum or menopausal women. Dr. Joffe and his research team at the Perinatal and Reproductive Psychiatry Division of Harvard Medical School are working on a study that concentrates on the effects of estrogen on the central nervous system and on serotonin levels. Another study out of the Medical University of South Carolina has found that one of the major reasons women become more depressed than men is related to their changing hormone levels. They reported that estrogen not only alters serotonin activity in the brain, it also impacts the activity of several other neurotransmitters that control mood.

There are negative effects that can occur when estrogen levels in the body are high (see sidebar). If estrogen is properly balanced, however, with progesterone, these effects don't happen. If you take the pill, are pregnant, or about to have your period, however, estrogen levels can soar, creating a shortage of tryptophan or vitamin B6. The result is often drastic changes in mood and physical well-being. One of the benefits of taking extra vitamin B6 is that is has been shown to decrease estradiol (a type of estrogen) in the bloodstream. At the same time, it helps boost progesterone levels to normalize hormonal balance in the body.

Women who take synthetic estrogen (hormone replacement therapy) to relieve menopausal symptoms may also develop a vitamin B6 deficiency that contributes to a depressed mental state. Studies suggest that taking supplemental vitamin B6 may increase levels of serotonin and dopamine in the brain, thereby combating depression.

As someone who has battled hormonally driven mood slumps, I can relate to women who feel like they're losing their sanity every month. Dramatic fluctuations in mood and extreme irritability are common side effects of estrogen-stimulated disorders. Knowing that estrogen can alter normal brain biochemistry helps explain the emotional roller coaster a woman rides throughout her life.

ESTROGEN AND ELIMINATION

In addition to low levels of progesterone, other factors can also lead to estrogen dominance. When it comes to dangerous estradiol levels, poor elimination poses a threat most women aren't aware of. A significant amount of estrogen is excreted in bowel movements as a way to promote hormone balance. If your colon is lazy or backed up and estrogen-laced waste sits in the bowel for twenty-four hours or more, estrogen can be reabsorbed back into the body. When this happens, the liver and other organs—like the brain—are influenced by more estrogen exposure. Not only can this effect hurt women emotionally, excess estrogen exposure can increase the risk of breast and uterine cancers.

A Tuft's University study found that lower blood estrogen levels correlated with heavier stool weight, suggesting that estrogen is continually eliminated through bowel movements. To illustrate this fact, consider that the widespread use of birth control pills and HRT has actually resulted in the synthetic estrogen pollution of many of our lakes and rivers by way of our sewage systems. (For more on the colon connection to depression, see Chapter 9.)

Women, Chocolate and Depression

Stress and hormones aren't the only factors that play a major role in female depression. Chocolate—a major coping food for the PMS female—can also cause mood problems. Americans ate nearly 12 pounds of chocolate per head in 1997, according to the U.S Department of Commerce. It is the single-most commonly craved food in America, especially among women. In fact, a recent study in the *Journal of the American Dietetic Association* reported that a chocolate craving is there for a good reason. Not only does it smell and taste good, it also has a real antidepressant effect. Chocolate is rich in fat, sugar, cocoa butter and caffeine—all of which impact brain chemistry.

Chocolate contains a compound called phenylethylamine that has been compared to the drug ecstasy. It also contains cannabinoid fatty acids similar to those found in marijuana. New studies tell us that women may experience intense chocolate cravings just prior to when their period begins because as progesterone levels rise, the body is prompted to increase fat storage. This may also explain why so many women crave greasy chips and cheeseburgers during pre-period days. The combination of fat and sugar is particularly appealing.

New studies now suggest that fat and sugar together create an endorphin-like effect in the brain that elevates mood and creates a feeling of well being. I don't know about you, but at certain times of the month you can find me rummaging through every drawer and cupboard in the house looking for anything chocolate. If there were ever a food that epitomizes the best of sugar/fat combinations, it has to be chocolate. Chocolate is comprised of 50 percent fat and 50 percent sugar, in addition to the phenylethylamine— similar to the amino acid phenylalanine that stimulates the release of pleasure—creating endorphins in the brain.

Anecdotal studies have suggested that frequently, women who suffer from depression consistently crave chocolate. The phenylethylamine content of chocolate also has amphetamine-like stimulant properties. The traditional association between chocolates and romance may be based on the feelings of well-being the phenylalanine creates. Low blood levels of phenylalanine and tyrosine have both been found in depressed patients. Anyone who suffers from PMS will probably tell you that their craving for chocolate almost becomes pathological. If you find yourself mixing up cocoa and sugar as a midafternoon snack, you may be low in phenylalanine.

More importantly, if you are low in phenylalanine, you may be susceptible to depression. The fact that chocolate acts as a temporary mood elevator may explain why so many women eat chocolate both before and during their menstrual periods. Other studies have also found that women who suffer from PMS can suffer from deficiencies of magnesium—also contained in chocolate.

Some experts have recommended that women indulge their chocolate cravings. If you're trying to avoid the caffeine in chocolate, you may want to try carob snacks. Carob candies, cookies and other foods are available at health food stores.

Carbohydrate Cravings and Estrogen

We've already talked about carbohydrate cravings and mood. New studies have also found that the sugar cravings many women experience during PMS, pregnancy or menopause could be a response to the effect that estrogen has on both brain chemicals and blood sugar levels. Moreover, there is some evidence that women are more sensitive to serotonin fluctuations than men. Some experts believe that when estrogen levels fall and progesterone levels are high, serotonin levels may dip. (Again, we see a hormonal extreme here.)

Both high and low estrogen levels seem to impact brain chemistry, and when serotonin levels decrease, carbohydrate cravings are created. The same scenario can occur during perimenopause, or the years just prior to menopause. This may be one reason why menopausal women have a tendency to gain weight. Lower estrogen equals lower serotonin and an increased appetite for carbohydrates. More times than not, that craving is satisfied with foods replete with fatty carbohydrates, such as potato chips, cookies, or candy bars. Some nutritionists believe that women could avoid the pitfalls of PMS and other related estrogen problems if they kept their body supplied with ample nutrients.

Incidentally, Pamela Morford, M.D., a gynecologist in Minneapolis, has said, "The premenstrual problems of at least ninety percent of my patients can be traced to chronic candidiasis (a yeast infection). I have found that when I give these patients anti-candida therapy, they get better." For more information on the link between mood disorders and candidiasis, see Chapter 13.

Vitamin B6 and L-Tryptophan for PMS Mood Slumps

I have mentioned before that a deficiency of vitamin B6 can cause PMS symptoms, including depression, and it is linked to mood. In fact, some researchers speculate that many health problems—including mood disorders—can be linked to nutrient deficiencies. When it comes to counteracting hormonal stress, you may have to go well beyond the RDA for your vitamin and mineral supplementation. According to Alan Gaby, M.D., taking 50 mg of vitamin B6 daily can significantly control the low moods and other symptoms that accompany PMS. This is twenty-five times the RDA for vitamin B6. Recent studies support the use of vitamin B6 (up to 100 mg/day) for depression and other premenstrual symptoms.

In addition, a placebo-controlled clinical trial using L-tryptophan for premenstrual depression found that it helped to ease mood swings, tension and irritability by 34.5 percent as compared to 10.4 percent who took a placebo drug. The authors of the study concluded that tryptophan increased serotonin levels during certain points in the menstrual cycle, thereby helping to avoid the depression typically seen pre-period. L-tryptophan alone is not currently available for purchase; however, 5-HTP (5-hydroxytryptophan), which contains a metabolite of tryptophan, is on the market and is part of the core protocol plan for the treatment of depression.

Your Hormonal Havoc May Be Due to a Nutrient Deficiency Disorder

Physician Guy Abraham believes that malnutrition and stress underpin PMS. He strongly recommends that women should avoid caffeine, sugar, nicotine, alcohol, salt, fatty or fried foods, and excess dairy products. He advises a diet based on plenty of fresh fruits and vegetables, fish, legumes and whole grains. The fact that we eat meat from cattle and pigs that have been given estrogen-containing supplements to fatten them up quickly may also add to the problem of hormonal imbalances.

The Link Between Postpartum Depression and Vitamin B and Folic Acid Deficiencies

Zoltan P. Rona, a physician and author, points out that researchers have found that postpartum depression may be due to a lack of B-complex vitamins, calcium and magnesium. Rona goes on to emphasize that medical literature cites several cases of postpartum depression that were essentially cured in a week by using high folic acid supplementation and vitamin B12 injections. One study reported that out of eighteen women who were depressed the week after they had given birth, the ones who were the most severely depressed had the lowest tryptophan levels. (Remember that tryptophan makes serotonin.)

An article from *American Journal of Obstetrics and Gynecology* relates a case in which a woman suffered from unusually serious postpartum depression. She became progressively worse during the weeks following the birth of her baby—so much so that she believed she might harm herself or her new baby. She was hospitalized in two different psychiatric institutions and received shock treatments and various drugs but showed no significant improvement and even tried to commit suicide three times. Eventually her folate levels were tested, and they were so low that one was labeled "undetectable." She was given five milligrams of folic acid twice a day, which is considered a mega-dose. After ten days, she experienced a complete turn around, was discharged and told to take one milligram of folic acid every day. (The RDA for folic acid is set at 400 mcg for pregnant women, an amount that is now considered too low by a number of doctors.)

Menopausal Mood Slumps

Menopause has a bad reputation when it comes to mood swings and depression. Beginning in their mid-forties, most women battle the estrogen-progesterone seesaw in what is now called perimenopause. Women who have never experienced any emotional problems may feel anxious, nervous, unable to sleep and depressed. As a woman starts menopause, her estrogen levels dramatically dip causing irregular periods, weight gain, headaches, hot flashes and related symptoms. To make matters worse, if a woman at this age is nutrient deficient, she lacks the amino acids, B vitamins or key minerals (like magnesium) that work to keep the brain in good condition.

There is some speculation that women who are estrogen-deficient are also low in a hormone called pregnenolone. This compound not only serves as a precursor to progesterone, but also contributes to nerve cell transmissions in the brain. Simply put, when estrogen levels diminish, the brain is affected and depression can result. By using natural phytoestrogens such as those found in soy isoflavones and in natural progesterone cream, the impact of menopause on mood can be significantly neutralized.

It is also interesting to note that just like estrogen in women, testosterone levels have also been linked to mood alterations in men. Men aged fifty to eighty-nine are more susceptible to depressed moods if their amount of free-circulating testosterone is low. A new study suggests that testosterone treatment for these men might improve depressed mood (especially in older individuals).

Supplement Game Plan for Hormonally Driven Depression (Use with Core Protocol)

LIGHT THERAPY

Background information: A very interesting study published in 1999 found that light therapy—typically used to treat SAD (seasonal affective disorder)—may be beneficial for treating depression associated with PMS. The study reported that using active bright white light significantly reduced depression and premenstrual tension. In addition, light therapy has been used to help regulate menstrual periods in some women.

SOY ISOFLAVONES

Typical dosage: Natural phytoestrogens like the genistein and daidzein contained in soy can be of great benefit for women trying to achieve hormonal balance. Try to eat no less than 25 and no more than 60 grams of soy protein daily. While the isoflavone content of soy foods varies considerably for each product, one or two servings of tofu, soybeans or soy milk a day is equivalent to the normal soy intake of Asian women and includes approximately 35 mg of isoflavones. One cup of soybeans provides 300 mg of isoflavones.

NATURAL PROGESTERONE CREAMS

Typical dosage: These creams have natural compounds that are close in their chemical structure to progesterone and are absorbed through the skin. They can help balance estrogen levels, thereby easing PMS. Most women use one half teaspoon of the cream twice daily for the last two weeks of their cycle on vascular areas where veins are visible. If you want more information on natural progesterone creams, refer to books by Dr. John R. Lee, who is considered one of the foremost experts on using these creams for women's disorders.

CHASTE BERRY (VITEX AGNUS CASTUS)

Typical Dosage: Use a standardized product that contains 0.5 agnuside and take 175 to 225 mg daily. This herb acts on the pituitary gland to normalize hormonal function. Clinical evidence supports the traditional use of vitex in the treatment of PMS and menopausal complaints. German researchers conducted a controlled, double-blind study to evaluate the efficacy and safety of a standardized vitex supplement in comparison with pyridoxine (vitamin B6) in 175 women with PMS. Vitex was associated with a considerably better alleviation of typical PMS complaints, such as breast tenderness, edema, tension, headache, constipation and depression.

VITAMIN B6/B-COMPLEX
Note: This recommendation for a B-complex vitamin can replace the recommendation for B vitamins listed in the Core Protocol.

Background information: Taking extra vitamin B6 can treat water retention and mood swings that can occur during PMS or menopause, and B-complex vitamins may protect against some of the dangerous effects of estradiol and estrone in the body. Moreover, estrogen imbalances have been linked to a vitamin B6 deficiency.

CALCIUM
Note: The recommendation listed here can replace the recommendation for calcium supplementation listed in the Core Protocol.

Background information: Taking supplemental calcium resulted in a 50 percent reduction of PMS symptoms in one clinical study of 400 women. Dr. Susan Thys-Jacobs of St. Luke's-Roosevelt Hospital reported that mood swings, tension, headaches and cramping were all alleviated with calcium supplementation. Food cravings also dropped by half, and water retention decreased by more than one-third. Look for citrate products combined with magnesium.

Typical Dosage: Take 2,000 mg. daily.

VITAMIN E
Background information: Tests with vitamin E dramatically support its use for hot flashes and other menopausal symptoms. In

some tests, it also worked better than barbiturates to calm anxiety. While some controversial data surrounding the use of vitamin E and breast cancer exists, the overwhelming consensus is that this vitamin helps to prevent breast fibroids, reduces the risk of heart disease, and may help to ease hormonally-induced symptoms.

Vitamin C

Background information: Clinical studies of menopausal women also found that using vitamin C with hesperidin (a bioflavonoid) relieved symptoms in 50 percent of ninety-four women who participated in the study. Leg cramps, bruising and hot flashes also significantly decreased. Interestingly, certain bioflavonoids actually resemble estradiol in their chemical structure.

Note: All of these vitamins (and calcium) have been included in the core protocol for treating depression so you won't need to add these to your program for hormonally driven symptoms.

The Profound Value of Exercise for Emotional Problems Caused by Hormones

In addition to these supplements, the value of regular exercise for women of all ages cannot be overemphasized. I've heard women profess on more than one occasion that exercising has preserved their physical well being as well as saved their sanity. Exercising can help to neutralize hormonally induced miseries that characterize PMS and menopause. It can also ease crampy periods and stress created by the ebb and flow of hormones. Clinical studies have found that hot flashes are half as common in women who engage in regular physical activity. Additionally, entering menopause with strong bones and toned muscles can help women avoid osteoporosis. Burning calories also helps to maintain ideal body weight, which may become more difficult with each passing year, especially important when considering the dangers of excess weight on health. Did you know, for instance, that carrying extra weight can also contribute to hormonal imbalances? Fat cells make estrogen. The heavier you are, the more you likely you are to experience estrogen dominance. On the other hand, if a woman is too thin, she may experience more estrogen depletion than normal during menopause, which could make her symptoms worse.

Exercising regularly is also considered by many experts to be the most significant weapon against the negative psychological symptoms that often characterize PMS and menopause. I would also say that an active lifestyle should be a primary part of your depression treatment, especially depression related to hormone imbalances.

Engaging in some sort of aerobic workout (brisk walking, jogging, biking) three to five times a week for 30 to 45 minutes is recommended. Working out with weights is also good to build muscle mass and prevent osteoporosis. Weight-bearing exercises are particularly good to help maintain bone density. Also, as you continue to piece together your depression puzzle, keep a record of the effects that exercise has on your mood and other factors. It may be helpful when you are investigating other treatments.

CHAPTER 11

The Light Link to Mood

*Light is the first of painters. There is no object so foul that
intense light will not make it beautiful.*

RALPH WALDO EMERSON

ON MAY 16, 1898, arctic explorer Frederick A. Cook wrote in his
journal:

> The winter and the darkness have slowly but steadily settled over us.
> It is not difficult to read on the faces of my companions their thoughts
> and their moody dispositions. The curtain of blackness which has fall-
> en over the outer world of icy desolation has also descended upon the
> inner world of our souls. Around the tables, men are sitting about sad
> and dejected, lost in dreams of melancholy from which now and then,
> one arouses with an empty attempt at enthusiasm.

It has been estimated that up to 10 percent of the population
experiences what Cook just described—a condition called "winter
blues" or SAD (seasonal affective disorder). In fact, according to
the National Institute of Mental Health (NIMH), over ten million
Americans experience SAD every year, and another twenty-five
million become mildly depressed on a seasonal basis.

SAD is a form of depressive illness that tends to occur during
times of light deprivation. As we study SAD more, we begin to

appreciate the hundreds of biological or circadian rhythms that occur in our bodies over a 24-hour period, and how they impact our behavior and emotional state. All of these rhythms are determined by our internal clock. A hormone called melatonin is released according to the workings of our body clocks, influenced by the presence of light and darkness. Experts believe that we were designed to go to sleep when it gets dark and arise when sunlight appears. During the winter months, this scenario does not always hold true. Not only do we see less sunlight, but we also commonly get up when it's still dark outside. When we go against our natural body clocks, our biorhythms can become disrupted. As a result, we can experience sleep disorders, fatigue and depression.

Because seasonal changes and light exposure can affect our moods so dramatically, it is imperative that we consider these factors when puzzle-solving our depression. Our exposure to light actually manipulates hormones like melatonin and other brain neurotransmitters, and when we become light deprived, many of us also start to feel down in the dumps. If this only seems to occur during the winter months or in places where sunlight is rare, we may have a case of seasonal affective disorder, and like any other form of depression, the effects of SAD can be crippling. SAD can affect job performance and family relationships.

While most of us gripe more during the cold, dark months of winter, some of us actually become physically incapacitated. In addition, anyone struggling with SAD may overeat to compensate for low feelings, and the resulting weight gain only makes the problem worse.

Over the last ten years, studies have closely investigated the impact that a light deficiency has on certain individuals. More and more psychiatrists and endocrinologists are recognizing the complex effects that light exerts on the human body. What they have found is that a lack of light can cause the nervous system to become depressed.

This seasonal depression is somewhat different in its symptoms than classical depression. The main differences between people who suffer from SAD and other forms of depression is that SAD victims tend to eat more—turning to carbohydrates or alcohol for mental stimulation, and they frequently oversleep. While a loss of appetite and insomnia are the general rule in standard cases of depression, the opposite behaviors can occur in SAD. The fact that a seasonal change can clear up SAD also distinguishes it from standard depression. For a clinically depressed person, even the arrival of spring fails to exhilarate.

Light and Biochemistry

Along with its ability to elevate mood, light is believed to affect female ovulation and the ability of the body to absorb calcium. Light therapy is also used to treat jaundice in newborns. It is now believed that the number of daylight hours we are exposed to tells our bodies and minds what time of day and year it is. This explains, in part, why our appetites and sleep patterns vary. Light can stimulate or suppress the secretion of the hormones that regulate these cycles.

For example, the pineal gland produces a hormone called melatonin, which produces a desire to sleep in most animals. As the day darkens, the pineal gland begins to respond by producing melatonin. In addition, melatonin also raises the level of serotonin in the brain.

The Melatonin Mood Link

Some people with SAD also suffer from unusual disruptions in their melatonin cycles. Melatonin secretion typically increases during the winter months and usually peaks around midnight. Interestingly, melatonin secretion decreases in women during the summer months and remains relatively unchanged in men.

Our artificially lit or dim environments can confuse our melatonin cycles, creating abnormal sleep and mood patterns. If you've ever attended a lecture in a dimly lit classroom, you may have become overwhelmed by a sudden desire to sleep. Scientists think that the supply of light that enters the eye either stimulates or suppresses the release of melatonin. When morning light reaches the pineal gland through the eyes, melatonin production is stopped. It is for this reason that surgically removing the eyes of a totally blind person for cosmetic reasons is not advisable. Even blind eyes can respond to the presence of light. Because the pineal gland is interrelated with the rest of the endocrine system, its function affects the pituitary gland, which in turn affects the thyroid gland, the adrenal glands, etc.

So why do some of us still feel drowsy or lethargic in a brightly lit room? The reason we still get sleepy under artificial lights if it's late at night is that indoor lighting is not intense enough to trigger the hormonal responses needed to keep us awake. Research has shown that lights of at least 2,500 lux are required to suppress the production of melatonin, and the average electric light bulb is approximately 500 lux. Therefore, low intensity, artificial light does not satisfy our bodies' requirement for natural sunlight. Dr. Richard Wurtman points out that the artificial lights typically used to illuminate interiors provide only one-tenth of the light we would find outdoors under one shade tree on a sunny day.

It would seem then, that if daylight hours could be extended, a whole variety of mental and physical reactions would result. Studies have concluded that in several countries even the rate of conception increases when daylight hours are the longest. Exposure to sunlight has been found to impact the timing and quality of sleep, appetite fluctuations, sexual activity, the onset of the menstrual cycle, pain endurance, and mood.

How Does SAD Make You Feel?

People who suffer from SAD feel just that—sad, low, anxious and irritable. They may also be consistently fatigued and oversleep or fall asleep during the day. In addition, they usually crave sweets and junk food that make them gain weight. These sentiments are typical of one suffering from SAD:

> I just can't get up in the morning. Even with the Christmas season approaching, I can't seem to muster the energy I need to make the hol-

Symptoms of Seasonal Affective Disorder (SAD)

The following list is a summary of symptoms common to those suffering from seasonal affective disorder.

- aggravated premenstrual symptoms
- cravings for carbohydrates and sweets
- depression
- headaches
- irritability and inability to focus

- hypersomnia or increased sleep by as much as four or more hours per night and reduced quality of the sleep
- seasonal behavioral changes, particularly increased sleep and variations in appetite
- weight gain

idays special. I feel so tired and melancholy. All I want to do is get under the covers and sleep. When I'm not sleeping, I want to eat. First I'll eat some cookies, then I'll crave some ice cream, and then I'll want something salty like potato chips. I've gained weight and that makes me feel even worse. I don't want anybody to see me. I'm also having trouble concentrating and making even simple choices. I feel like a lazy slob but I can't seem to snap out of it.

SAD is characterized by comfort eating, fatigue and oversleeping, and keep in mind that the type of sleep SAD sufferers experience only serves to make them feel more tired. For this kind of depression, light starvation is the culprit.

Food Cravings and Light

During the winter months, serotonin levels in the brain can be at their lowest. Eating carbohydrates can boost serotonin levels, a simple fact that may explain why SAD victims crave carbohydrates. But that's not the whole story. It seems that exposure to bright light influences serotonin production, and to some extent, works in the same way as antidepressant drugs. Today, the general consensus is that SAD, like other mood disorders, may be initiated by biochemical disturbances. The role of melatonin and serotonin are vital to controlling mood and appetite and exposure to light manipulates these repetitive patterns in some people. What is particularly fascinating is that the classic symptoms of SAD are strikingly similar to women who get PMS, people who binge on carbohydrates and obese individuals. These symptoms include lethargy, overeating, weight gain, the inability to concentrate and depression. In all three of these disorders, symptoms occurred only during certain time intervals—for SAD, during dark, winter months, for PMS, just prior to the menstrual period and for carbohydrate cravers, during the late afternoon or evening hours. Studies tell us that carbohydrate cravers overeat only at certain times of the day. While calorie intake was normal at mealtime, snacking in the late afternoon or early evening dramatically increased caloric intake, and protein snacks are rarely chosen.

People with SAD eat the same way. One SAD victim expressed, "I eat to combat a feeling of mental fatigue." What researchers found was that exposing SAD patients to a few hours of sufficient light every morning could not only eliminate depression but their carbohydrate craving as well. In light of these findings (no pun intended) it has been suggested that obese individuals and women suffering from PMS may also benefit from light therapy.

Obviously, in all three of these groups, serotonin malfunctions trigger carbohydrate binging. Interestingly, some antidepressant drugs that manipulate serotonin have a tendency to suppress carbohydrate snacking and relieve depression. For this reason, drugs that boost serotonin neurotransmission (such as D-fenfluramine, femoxetine, fluoxetine, symelidine and fluvoxamine) have a tendency to promote weight loss, although this is not always the case. On the other hand, drugs that clock serotonin action or antidepressants that affect other neurotransmitters instead of serotonin can create carbohydrate cravings and weight gain.

Children and SAD

The effects of SAD on adults is well known, but it can also target children. In fact, many adults with SAD report that they commonly experienced winter blues as children and teenagers. A new study, published in the October issue of the *Journal of the American Academy of Child and Adolescent Psychiatry,* reports that as many as 60 to 90 percent of boys and girls report seasonal variations in energy, mood, length of sleep, and social activity. Feelings of lethargy and unexplained sadness are typical in the winter months and seem to disappear with the coming of spring. It's important to be aware that your child or teenager may be prone to SAD—a fact that may give you a much better understanding of their seemingly strange behavior. Because so much of the school year typically takes place during the winter months, you may want to look into light box therapy for your child in order to enhance school performance. Some experts believe that using light therapy in the morning can help to avoid troublesome behavior and fatigue later in the day.

Light Exposure and Vitamin D

Light exposure affects more than melatonin production and sleeping patterns. Without sunlight, our bodies cannot produce sufficient amounts of vitamin D. As a result of a vitamin D deficiency, calcium cannot be adequately absorbed into the bones and teeth. While some foods provide vitamin D, studies have shown that these sources are not as biologically effective as the vitamin D produced in the skin from sunlight exposure. I have noticed that even our dog Emerson finds the only patch of sunlight we get in our northern exposure home and makes sure he gets his daily sunbath. Incidentally, there is some speculation that the presence of smog in urban areas can inhibit the efficiency of ultraviolet light rays, impacting mood and vitamin D absorption.

A study of elderly men living in a nursing home in Boston found that when these men were isolated from natural daylight for seven weeks and exposed to only fluorescent or incandescent light, their calcium absorption was significantly impaired, due to a drop in vitamin D levels. It would be interesting to see if a drop in mood also corresponded to this sunlight deprivation.

Again, many elderly people who are confined to poorly lit interiors suffer from serious depression. Also, over the last twenty years, the availability of outdoor porches and verandas in convalescent homes has decreased. Sadly, most windows in professional care facilities don't even open.

Light Therapy is the Answer

A team of psychiatrists at the National Institute of Mental Health, in Bethesda, Maryland took thirty people with a history of winter depression and used light therapy (phototherapy) to treat them. Preliminary findings showed that using a special artificial light that mimics the light spectrum of the sun is very beneficial. This light reproduces the same effect seen on the longest day of the year. These people used the lights during the winter months for three hours every morning and every night with dramatic positive response.

Researchers have come away from studies such as this one believing that people with SAD could greatly benefit by doing something as simple as morning exposure to bright light. Interestingly, light exposure may also benefit people with other mental illnesses. Thomas Wehr and Norman Rosenthal, two medical doctors at the National Institute of Mental Health created an artificial "spring" as treatment for a 63-year-old manic-depressive patient. During the first week of December, they woke him up at 6:00 AM and exposed him to extremely bright artificial light for three hours. At 4:00 PM, they repeated the exposure for another three hours. Simply stated, they artificially lengthened his days. They continued this therapy for ten days. After only four days, this man felt much better and began to come out of his social withdrawal.

USING A LIGHT BOX

To combat SAD, use a light box of up to 10,000 lux that can use either fluorescent tubes or full-spectrum lighting. These boxes are designed for placement at a table and can be tilted to maximize exposure. Ultraviolet rays have been screened out of these lights to prevent injury to skin and eyes. You don't have to use sunscreen when using these boxes, either. Full-spectrum light bulbs resemble natural sunlight more closely than do fluorescent or regular light bulbs.

If you have SAD, you should start to see an improvement within the first few days of light therapy. If you're not sure you have SAD, try the box on a trial basis before you invest the money to purchase one. There are over 10,000 of these light boxes in use today. Portable light dosage systems are also available. Keep in mind that treatments typically last for at least thirty minutes a day at 10,000 lux (twenty times normal indoor lighting).

Morning Light Exposure May Be Best

One study of ninety-six SAD patients conducted at the Rush-Presbyterian-St. Luke's Medical Center in Chicago found that 61 percent of people exposed to morning light therapy and 50 percent of people who received evening light therapy experienced nearly complete recovery from their seasonal depression after four weeks of treatment. Researchers at Oregon Health Sciences University in Portland compared the effectiveness of morning to evening light therapy as well. They discovered that morning therapy is at least twice as effective as evening therapy.

One theory proposes that bright lights suppress the brain's secretion of melatonin, which wakes us up. Data reveals that in approximately 80 percent of people with SAD, melatonin levels peak when it's time to wake up. Light therapy helps to reverse this trend. If you are one of those people who typically wake up in the middle of the night, evening light therapy may be a better choice for you.

Other Interesting Facts about Light Therapy

The average light box costs between $200 and $400. If you think this is too expensive, consider the overall cost of prescription drugs and psychotherapy. Preliminary research has shown that these light boxes help up to 85 percent of people suffering from SAD. If you can't afford a light box, ask your doctor if he has one, or if he knows of one that can be rented.

And what about the possible value of light therapy for other forms of depression? Some psychiatrists have suggested that phototherapy may be of value in treating nonseasonal depression as well. There is evidence that exposing depressed individuals to bright light may be as effective in reducing some types of depression as antidepressant drugs. The studies done by the Wurtmans certainly suggest that light may be a more significant piece of the puzzle in disorders such as PMS and obesity than previously thought.

In the meantime, if you suffer from any kind of depression, provide your environment with sufficient light and invest in a light box if you think it might help. Consider putting in a skylight as well. The following are other recommendations to provide an optimal environment for battling depression.

- Make your environment as light accessible as possible.
- Place reading chairs and desktops near windows.
- Keep your curtains drawn back or invest in lightweight shades or blinds that don't block out light.
- Don't clutter window sills or place furniture in front of light sources.
- Use light colored paints and upholstery, and purchase track lighting that can be added to your existing ceiling light fixture.
- Keep your home well ventilated with fresh air.
- Bring colorful plants and flowers into your environment.
- For those of you who live in agreeable climates, make sure you get out in the sun every day for at least a couple of hours (though it is a good idea to check with your doctor before initiating any kind of light therapy).

• If you suffer from certain eye conditions or skin disorders, phototherapy should not be used.

For more information on treating SAD, contact the National Organization for SAD: P.O. Box 40133, Washington, DC 20016.

Supplement Game Plan for SAD (Use with Core Protocol)

LIGHT THERAPY

Background information: Use full-spectrum light therapy, such as Vita-Lite, and stay within the light's rays for approximately three hours in the early morning and three hours in the early evening. Then adjust down exposure as needed. You may find that you do not need both morning and evening exposure.

VITAMIN **D**

Typical dosage: 400 IU daily of the vitamin D3 form

A NOTE ON USING SUPPLEMENTAL MELATONIN

While some experts recommend melatonin for SAD, I have found that using it can worsen depressive symptoms. For this reason, I don't recommend its use for those who are susceptible to depression.

CHAPTER 12

Sleep Disorders and Mood

The average, healthy, well-adjusted adult gets up at seven-thirty
in the morning feeling just plain terrible.
JEAN KERR

CLEARLY, AN INTIMATE relationship exists between depression and sleep, whether it be too much or too little sleep. And despite the fact that we sleep for almost half of our lives, sleep and its relationship to our overall health has been surprisingly neglected by physicians and scientists. In fact, it's only been within the last two decades that the effects of sleep (or a lack of it) have been addressed. Evidence supports that any alteration in healthy sleep patterns can throw us into a depressive state. It is also true that if you're depressed, you probably have trouble sleeping.

Four out of five people who become depressed view bedtime with dread. What should be a time for rest and rejuvenation can turn into a tortuous period of tossing and turning, characterized by obsessive, negative thoughts. The simple ability to relax and fall asleep peacefully can become almost impossible for depressed individuals. Moreover, even if they get to sleep, they frequently awake and fill their minds with distressing and troubling thoughts.

What do depressed people think about? Anything and everything that is gloomy, scary or self-defeating. I have had some experience with this type of troubled sleep. I will sometimes wake up at around three in the morning and begin to worry about money, earthquakes, getting fat, being alone, comets hitting the earth, if I might have cancer, my children's happiness, and so on. When this happens, sleep vanishes and anxiety slips in, often keeping me awake until the early morning hours. If I do get some predawn rest, it's minimal and I wake up feeling exhausted and grumpy.

You'll probably agree that these kinds of thought patterns are common during periods of sleeplessness and usually aren't based on reality. As most of you know, lying in the dark can intensify fearful and apprehensive feelings and make everything seem a hundred times worse than it really is. Thankfully, the arrival of day helps to dispel many of our night terrors. On the other hand, in cases of severe depression, the torture can continue.

Since the amount and kind of sleep you are getting can affect your mood so completely, it is important to spend time puzzle-solving the role sleep has in your life and in your depression, whether you are occasionally or consistently suffering through sleep disturbances. By carefully analyzing your sleeping habits, the kinds of rest you are getting, the times of day you feel fatigued and why, as well as other factors, you may solve a significant portion of your depression puzzle.

All Sleep Isn't Necessarily Good Sleep

Undoubtedly, sleep disturbances can cause depressive illness or result from its presence. Some scientists believe that the wrong kind of sleep initiates depression. They suggest that the chemical changes that occur in the brain during sleep may have a direct bearing on the nerves and neurotransmitters that produce depression. Perhaps this explains the existence of "morning people." Surely there must be a biological reason why some of us wake up grumpy, moody and irritable, while others are prone to singing and whistling. The notion that sleeping by itself may not be enough to promote a good mood is worth investigating. Perhaps the kind of sleep we get is just as important as how long we sleep.

Most people who feel depressed not only experience shortened intervals of sleep, but also poor quality sleep.

We all know that a bad night's sleep can impair alertness and result in all kinds of accidents. Some experts believe that Americans operate on a sleep deficit, which is the real reason for the erratic behavior we see all around us. Most of us go to bed too late and sleep poorly, or we take hypnotic drugs to get to sleep and stimulants to wake up. In a study on sleep deprivation, 40 percent of the subjects tested were found to be "pathologically sleepy" during the day.

Clearly, much of the evidence in this book supports the fact that disturbed brain biochemistry can be responsible for nighttime as well as daytime mind-sets. Nonrestful sleep can make us feel as if we haven't slept at all, and although sleep disorders are common, they should not be considered normal. In fact, they almost always signal the presence of another problem. This is especially true for depression.

REM Sleep and Depressive Illness

Some studies have shown that by depriving a person of rapid eye movement (REM) sleep for an extended period of time, various psychotic conditions result, including severe depressive illness. REM sleep is the stage of sleep when we dream and do a great deal of cellular repair and regeneration. One reason why we feel so emotionally shot when we don't sleep well is because the cells of the nervous system are rebuilt during REM sleep. If you lack REM sleep, protein production in the brain is inhibited, preventing the normal restoration of cells required to keep us mentally healthy.

We need a certain amount of REM sleep to feel happy and healthy. Ironically, many drugs—some of which are used to help induce sleep or counteract depression—can actually interfere with or diminish REM sleep. To make matters even more confusing, disrupted sleep can cause depression, and depression can cause disrupted sleep. Solving the puzzle of which came first can prove difficult. In any event, just knowing that serotonin levels are so crucial to proper REM sleep provides new insight into sleep and its intrinsic relationship with depression. Studies suggest that many depressed individuals tend to enter REM sleep more rapidly than normal and then leave it prematurely. This particular phenomenon is also typical of people suffering from schizophrenia, anorexia, mania and obsessive-compulsive disorders. Interestingly, a whole host of psychiatric diseases seem linked to disturbed sleep patterns. Dementia causes decreased delta waves during sleep, and panic disorders produce continually interrupted and decreased sleep. What research findings suggest is that if you're suffering from depression, even when you do sleep, you may not be experiencing true rest. Disruptions in REM sleep are a marker of behavioral disorders and a large piece in the depression puzzle.

Be aware also that a continual lack of quality sleep can actually accumulate over time. This sleep debt can result in subtle, unexplained symptoms. Interrupting the way the brain normally falls asleep, stays asleep and wakes up can create a sleep deficit. In addition, if you take any kind of drug, you may be significantly compromising the quality of your sleep. Sedatives, stimulants like caffeine, anticonvulsants and antihistamines are just a few of the many chemical agents that interfere with normal sleep patterns causing daytime fatigue. It's also important to know that if you are withdrawing from any of these drugs, your sleep may be altered for several weeks as your body adjusts to the absence of these chemical agents from the bloodstream.

Sleep disruption is like depression in that it can be initiated by so many hidden factors. For instance, smoking and obesity can affect respiration, which can result in sleep apnea. Sleep apnea refers to a condition of abnormal breathing or snoring that can actually deprive brain cells from adequate oxygen. A repeated lack of oxygen to brain tissue can result in mental fogginess, forgetfulness or emotional stupor. Exposure to polluted air, water, certain organic compounds, and heavy metals can also alter normal sleep. In addition, food allergies are notorious for causing insomnia or restless sleep, especially in children.

Serotonin, Sleep and Depression

At this point the "S" word comes up once again—serotonin not only assists in initiating REM sleep, but also has to be present in certain levels to adequately maintain REM sleep. Scientists have recently concluded that serotonin levels determine sleeping and waking cycles. This fact alone explains to some degree why sleeping habits and mood are so tightly interwoven. If you don't make or utilize enough serotonin, you may sleep for shorter intervals or not at all.

It also may be of interest to mention the use of tryptophan to induce sleep. Before it was taken off the market, tryptophan was successfully used to treat insomnia. The fact that tryptophan is a precursor to serotonin, which also helps to define our moods and attitudes, is no coincidence. It also points out that when we artificially manipulate serotonin through chemical agents, we can change sleep patterns.

It's rather fascinating that antidepressant drugs of the SSRI variety like Prozac actually inhibit REM sleep due to their unnatural action on serotonin levels. A common side effect of Prozac is the inability to sleep well. However, 5-HTP (5-hydroxytryptophan) is often recommended for disturbed sleep (as well as depression) and has replaced the tryptophan supplements that are no longer available. Unfortunately, many doctors readily prescribe sedative drugs to treat depressive insomnia—a practice that may actually perpetuate the disease.

Hypersomnia: Too Much of a Good Thing?

While it's typical for depressed people to sleep poorly, some people with melancholia have trouble with oversleeping. Hypersomnia refers to the need for more than a normal amount of sleep and can also occur when you feel depressed, especially in seasonal mood disorders. For more information regarding hypersomnia, see Chapter 11. Some people who feel depressed sleep to escape reality and pain. Going to bed offers a refuge

Hypnotic Drugs and Artificial Sleep

The scenario goes something like this: You can't sleep, so you take a sleeping pill, which disrupts your normal sleep patterns by suppressing REM sleep. Because you were cheated of REM sleep, you wake up more tired than you were before you went to sleep. To make matters worse, you try to solve the problem by not taking these pills after long-term use. However, you begin to experience severe withdrawal symptoms, including anxiety, seizures, hallucinations, panic, insomnia, memory loss and worsened depression. So, you begin to once again take the sleeping pills.

Every year, up to ten million people in this country use prescription drugs to get to sleep. Benzodiazepines (one class of sleeping pills) can produce a variety of undesirable side effects, including lethargy, amnesia, memory impairment, nervousness and aggressiveness. These drugs act on brain chemistry, therefore affecting behavior. I would think it safe to assume that even if you're depressed and suffering from insomnia, one of the worst things you could do to yourself is to add benzodiazepines to your system. This family of hypnotic drugs, which includes Halcion, Valium, Librium, Ativan, Dalmane and Clonopin, to mention only a few, has been shown to worsen feelings of depression and may even prompt suicidal thinking.

If you have trouble sleeping, make an effort to forgo the drug route and concentrate on relaxation techniques and natural therapies. If possible, avoid the temptation to use sedatives or other sleep-promoting drugs. Most of them are addictive and only serve to make you feel hung over and more depressed. Before you initiate the vicious cycle of artificial sedation, try relaxation techniques, dietary changes and natural supplements (listed at the end of this chapter).

from the world that reminds us how worthless we feel. Keep in mind that getting too much sleep can make you feel as unrested as getting too little. Our biological clocks usually determine the optimal amount of sleep we need to feel good. When we sleep too little or too much, that clock becomes skewed, and nine times out of ten, it's due to a neurochemical disruption. The way we wake up from a night's sleep can also impact our mental attitude for the day.

A Kinder, Gentler Waking

Deepak Chopra, M.D., in his book *Quantum Healing*, tells us that human beings need to wake up from sleep through a series of timed signals that progress from mild to strong. He stresses that ideally, to go from the biochemistry of sleep to the biochemistry of wakefulness, the transition should be gradual. However, most of us are abruptly woken out of a dead sleep by a blaring alarm that jars our brains out of its state of rest. Remember that if you wake up in the middle of your sleep cycle and disrupt the normal pattern of sleep, you can feel groggy, moody and irritable during the day.

Use a gentle alarm system that wakes you up in multiple increments of time. As you awake, slowly stretch your body and take a number of deep breaths. As you rise, sit on the side of your bed and rest for a moment before getting completely out. This would be an optimal time to meditate or pray. Immediately let the sunshine in or turn on lights and then before you get dressed, try to do some form of limited exercise.

Programmed Sleeplessness: A Surprising Treatment for Depression

Another solution to sleep disorders may even be sleeplessness. As mentioned earlier, many depressed people take sleeping pills along with their antidepressant drugs. Why? First, many antidepressant drugs cause insomnia and agitation, and second, depression itself disrupts normal sleep patterns. While insomnia is thought to worsen depression, new data from a five-year study suggests that in some cases, preventing a person from sleeping actually boosts mood. In an article published in recent issue of the *American Journal of Psychiatry,* researchers reported that lack of sleep increased brain activity and decreased clinical depression in one third of the depressed patients studied. While this effect was dramatic, keep in mind that it was also very short lived. Another study found that depressed patients who benefited from sleep deprivation suffered a relapse after one night of sleep or even after taking a nap.

Sleep deprivation did not work for all of the depressed individuals tested, and for those individuals it did help with, it should not be used as a continual therapy due to its negative side effects. Its real value comes from gaining new insight into yet another link between the brain's mechanisms and mood control. What these studies imply is that for some people sleep itself acts as a depressant. Let's briefly describe sleep deprivation as a treatment for depressive illness.

SLEEP DEPRIVATION AS AN ANTIDEPRESSANT THERAPY

Sleep deprivation is still considered controversial. Remember that this sleep prohibition does not refer to random sleep that continually inhibits REM sleep; it is controlled and individually programmed. This particular treatment assumes that depression has a tendency to put the brain to sleep in an unnatural way. By programming periods of wakefulness, the brain, in some instances, become stimulated enough to sustain mood.

Some new studies at the National Institute of Mental Health in Bethesda, Maryland, have found that this technique works on the principle that keeping a person awake may serve to snap them out of a depressive state. Some doctors have suggested that sleep deprivation may hold promise as a supplemental treatment for those people who don't respond as they should to medication.

For instance, in 1993, researchers at the University Of Michigan's Adolescent Psychiatry Department deprived seventeen patients of sleep for thirty-six hours. They found that the severely depressed patients experienced significant relief in symptoms after staying awake; however, the patients who had been recovering from depression and those who were not depressed, experienced a mood slump. But for some people, staying up proved a much more effective treatment for their depression than drugs.

Surprisingly, these studies have found that staying up all night for these individuals promotes cheerfulness, conversation and light-hearted feelings, even in seriously depressed people. Because illness returns when these individuals resume their normal sleeping patterns, a system of partial sleep in which patients intersperse nights where they sleep for only five hours with normal sleeping hours has been recommended.

Interestingly, one theory as to why this works with certain people is that sleep deprivation stimulates the release of a compound called TSH that steps up the activity of a sluggish thyroid gland. The profound connection between inadequate amounts of thyroid hormone and depression are addressed in Chapter 13. A controlled lack of sleep can actually help to restore the adrenal hormone (cortisol) and TSH to normal levels, thereby improving mood. I would assume that if you feel better when you sleep less, you should have your thyroid gland checked.

PARTIAL SLEEP: A COMPROMISE

Partial sleep deprivation therapy has worked for 60 percent of patients suffering from major depression and involves cutting down periods of sleeplessness or alternating nights of full sleep with ones of partial sleep. It must be stressed here that this type of treatment is not for everyone suffering from depression and should only be done under the supervision of an expert. Sleep deprivation can be dangerous and can make depression worse if not done correctly.

Interestingly, some doctors have used sleep deprivation to prevent depression in people who suffer from periodic bouts of depression. This treatment involves staying up for 36 hours once a week and should be done only under the care of a doctor or health practitioner. Why sleep deprivation works when antidepressant drugs fail in some people is yet to be understood. Like other natural therapies, no significant side effects have been observed from this therapy; nevertheless, you need to find out if you're a candidate for this radical form of treatment before attempting it in any way.

The connection between sleep and depression is yet another piece of the puzzle. It reveals that brain biochemistry and behavior not only depend on how we eat, but how we sleep as well. If you want more information on the partial-sleep program contact Dr. Thomas Wehr and Dr. David A. Sack at the National Institute of Mental Health, in Bethesda, Maryland.

Regardless of whether you're undersleeping or oversleeping, if your depression continues to worsen, your sleeping disorders will only get worse. On the other hand, sleep improvement is often the first sign that your depression is lifting. As you get well, you will fall asleep faster and begin to sleep throughout the night. In conjunction with better sleep, your appetite will improve, and your spirits will rise. Each positive biochemical change initiates another.

Supplement Game Plan for Sleep Disorders (Use with Core Protocol)

VALERIAN ROOT
Typical dosage: Take 300 to 500 mg taken thirty minutes before bedtime. Look for products with a 0.8 percent valerenic acid content. Compounds found in this herb interact with brain receptor sites to promote better sleep patterns. There are literally dozens of pharmaceutical and tea forms of valerian used in Europe for sleep problems. Don't confuse valerian with the popular drug Valium, however, as they are not related in any way.

PASSION FLOWER
Typical dosage: This herb is widely used in Europe as a sedative. It also used to treat common nervous conditions like restlessness. 300 to 400 mg taken thirty minutes before bedtime. Taking this with your 5-HTP supplement (recommended in the core proto-

col for depression) may yield better results. Look for products with a 2.6 percent flavonoid content.

Kava Kava Root

Typical dosage: This herb has natural muscle-relaxant properties and has been used traditionally in the South Pacific to safely induce sleep. Take 45 to 70 mg kavalactones (also known as kavapyrones) thirty minutes before bedtime. Kava kava dosages depend on the kavalactone content of your kava kava root supplement. The content should be at least 3.5 percent kavalactones. Do not exceed recommended doses or combine with benzodiazepine drugs.

Suanzaorentang

Typical dosage: Take as directed. This Chinese herbal combination has been tested in double-blind studies and may help to treat not only insomnia, but actually improve daytime performance and alertness as well. Unlike the prescription drug diazepam (Valium), it did not result in feelings of irritability, depression or anxiety the next day. This combination of five herbs actually promotes a sense of well-being.

GABA (gamma aminobutyric acid)

Typical dosage: Take 200 to 400 mg thirty minutes before bedtime. GABA is an amino acid derivative.

Dietary Guidelines for Improved Sleep

Don't eat too close to bedtime because low blood sugar can be a contributing factor to insomnia. However, you may eat a piece of cheese with a whole-wheat cracker before retiring. Foods high in tryptophan also have a calming effect on the brain and include bananas, turkey, figs, tuna, dates, yogurt and milk. Avoid eating highly spiced foods, chocolate, smoked meats, sauerkraut and tomatoes too close to bedtime. There is some speculation that

Tips to Promote Optimal Sleep

• A bedtime snack is often helpful. The traditional home remedy of drinking a warm glass of milk has a scientific basis. Milk contains L-tryptophan that does help to induce sleep.

• A white noise machine emits a sound that masks other sounds and can help lull a person to sleep. A fish aquarium filter can produce the same effect.

• An outside stroll prior to bedtime is often helpful.

• Avoid drinking alcohol, especially in the evening. Alcohol can temporarily induce sleep; however, waking up in the middle of the night after a nightcap is common.

• Don't eat a large meal prior to bedtime. Not only can this result in insomnia, it can cause nightmares as well.

• Don't use nicotine. Smokers have more difficulty getting to sleep, according to researchers.

• Eliminate any over-the-counter or prescription drugs you do not need to take. Barbiturates and benzodiazepines can actively interfere with the sleep cycle.

• Exercise regularly. The value of exercise in enabling the body to relax at night cannot be overestimated. Exercise earlier in the day and not too close to bedtime. Twenty to thirty minutes of aerobic exercise at least three days a week is recommended.

• Get a pillow that is not too high or puffy. Feather pillows that compress down or special pillows designed to support your neck may be much more comfortable.

• Go to bed at the same time every night to establish a sleeping and waking routine for the body.

• If you can't sleep, get up. Read until you feel sleepy.

• Make sure your bedroom is well ventilated and not too hot.

• Never sleep in what you wore during the day. Use a light pajama or nightgown that is not too constricting or heavy.

• Once in bed, do breathing exercises while gently stretching your

---

> ## Tips to Promote Optimal Sleep (cont.)
>
> ▅
>
> limbs. Listening to a stress reducing tape that plays the sound of rain falling or ocean waves may also be helpful.
> * Relax and unwind before you go to bed by reading, listening to music or taking a bath.
> * Some people sleep better with an electric blanket or hot water bottle.
> * Switch to pure cotton or linen sheets if you don't use them already. Often the fabric that comes in contact with our skin can cause a subconscious annoyance.
> * Try to keep the bedroom as tranquil as possible, making it a place exclusively for sleep rather than other activities. Keep noise low and if necessary, purchase curtains that effectively block out light.
> * Yoga has been an effective meditative technique for combating insomnia.

these foods stimulate a release of norepinephrine, a brain stimulant. An effective, traditional nightcap for insomnia used in Spain is made by mixing two tablespoons of honey and the juice of one lemon in a glass of buttermilk.

Supportive Therapies

Aromatherapy. A warm bath scented with a few drops of essential oils, such as lavender, meadowsweet or orange blossom, will soothe the body and mind. Herbal baths can be quite relaxing and can be made by filling a muslin bag with herbs like lavender and attaching it to the faucet so hot water runs through it as the tub fills.

Homeopathy. *Aconite* is used for insomnia caused by fear, *Arnica* if you are overtired, and coffee for the racing mind. *Phosphorus* is also prescribed for nightmares, and *Nux vomica* for insomnia caused by alcohol consumption.

Massage. Hot oil massages can do more to relax a tense body than perhaps any other therapy. Try mixing one or two essential oils with olive or almond oil for massage.

Relaxation therapies. Mediation and yoga can initiate relaxation and free your mind from anxiety.

CHAPTER 13

Other Triggers of Depression

Quit worrying about your health. It'll go away.
ROBERT ORBEN

IN THIS BOOK, I have tried to show how many depressed people are suffering from a biological malfunction rather than a psychological one. In other words, this book has endeavored to prove that virtually any illness or disruption in our biology can initiate brain changes that make us feel blue. For example, yeast infections, fibromyalgia, thyroid disease and even cholesterol levels may cause you to become depressed. Yes, you read correctly—cholesterol levels can cause depression. According to a study reported in the November 1992 *Annals of Internal Medicine,* people who lowered their cholesterol over a five-year study period, also experienced a reduction in depression and hostility.

Of equal interest is the fact that women who suffer unexplained depression may have low thyroid function (hypothyroidism). Statistics tell us that up to 20 percent of people with depression have a sluggish thyroid. Immune dysfunction and stress are also major players in depressive disease. Interestingly, even if your depression is the result of a sad event, it is possible to set into motion biological cycles that perpetuate depression by increasing the body's susceptibility to it.

We're learning that even viruses can cause depression. Chronic fatigue syndrome, for example, is a disease caused by the Epstein-Barr virus and is considered a contributing factor to clinical depression. Fungi can also be culprits. Dr. Orian Truss, M.D., of Birmingham was one of the first doctors to recognize that depression can be a side effect of a chronic yeast infection that often targets women with compromised immunity. And then of course, there's fibromyalgia—a little understood but widespread, muscle-related disorder among women that also comes with a high incidence of prolonged periods of depression. In fact, fibromyalgia has recently been linked to serotonin dysfunction.

Other biological conditions that can cause unexplained depression include food allergies, irritable bowel syndrome, constipation, sleep disorders and hormonal imbalances. One psychiatrist explained that physical illnesses can produce systemic imbalances that may lead to profound emotional and mental changes. He goes on to say that many people who come to him with psychiatric symptoms have physical problems at the root of their mental disorders. He singles out allergies, viral infections, malnutrition and endocrine disorders, and he points out that as soon as these conditions are treated, the psychological symptoms clear up.

Singling out certain physical disturbances as causes for your depression can seem daunting. However, by applying a puzzle-solving approach, you have a system for careful evaluation that is far more effective than random testing. The rest of this chapter is dedicated to helping you apply this system. Each section describes an ailment that can cause mood disorders as well as symptoms, treatments and how the ailment affects brain chemistry and other mood-related factors.

Blame the Body

Although many sufferers of unexplained depression assume that their condition is the result of a character flaw or a punishment for not measuring up, often the cause of depression is much more physical. The real culprit can be chronic yeast infections, an inactive thyroid, or hidden food allergies. The good news is that when you treat any of these disorders—including depression—with natural medicine, you will inevitably improve your overall health as well.

Let's look into some of the more common (and often unrecognized) biological causes of depression. I will address those physical conditions that routinely predispose a person to depression. In each and every instance, the delicate balance of the brain's neurochemistry is altered. At the end of each discussion, a treatment plan is offered that should be combined with the core protocol for depression.

The Thyroid Connection to Depression

Low thyroid function and depressive illness are intimately connected. Because the function of brain amines or neurotransmitters interrelates with the endocrine system, people who are depressed frequently suffer from other hormonal malfunctions.

The hypothalamus is the area in the brain that regulates and balances your body's hormones. Like other brain tissue, it will respond to the chemical environment of the brain, producing the necessary hormones. In order to produce these hormones, it must be supplied with amino acids, essential fatty acids, and the appropriate vitamins and minerals.

Depression is often the first symptom of thyroid disease. Even a very subtle decrease in thyroid hormone can produce symptoms of depressive illness. Low thyroid function is referred to as hypothyroidism. Almost half of all people who suffer from an inactive thyroid also feel depressed.

SYMPTOMS OF AN UNDERACTIVE THYROID GLAND

Typically, anyone who has an underactive thyroid will feel chronically tired and will be unable to get things done at a normal pace. Mornings are particularly difficult due to a lack of energy.

Physical Conditions that Impact Brain Chemistry

Listed below are health conditions that may contribute to the onset of or worsening of depression:

- AIDS
- Addison's disease
- anemia (including pernicious anemia)
- cancer
- chronic fatigue syndrome
- constipation
- Crohn's disease
- Cushing's disease
- dementia (including Alzheimer's disease)
- endocrine disorders (such as hypothyroidism)
- epilepsy (temporal lobe)
- fibromyalgia
- food allergies
- Huntington's disease
- hypoglycemia
- immune system disorders
- influenza
- irritable bowel syndrome
- lupus erythematosus, systemic
- mononucleosis
- multiple sclerosis
- porphyria, intermittent
- stroke
- syphilis
- vitamin deficiencies (especially folic acid and vitamins B6 and B12)
- yeast infections

Other symptoms include:

- constipation
- dry, coarse skin
- excessive sleepiness
- hair loss
- hoarseness
- intolerance to cold/low basal temperature
- lack of perspiration
- menstrual cycle changes
- muscle weakness
- weight gain characterized by swelling and puffy tissues

If you suspect that you might have a thyroid problem, see your doctor. Keep in mind that a hypoactive thyroid is not easily diagnosed with designated lab tests. If you have any of the above symptoms in combination with chronic depression, you should suspect a sluggish thyroid. Request T3, T4 and TSH tests. If these are inconclusive, have your doctor run a TRH test as well.

THE THYROID, TYROSINE AND BRAIN CHEMICALS

In order for the thyroid gland to manufacture the hormone tyrosine, an amino acid and iodine are required. Some experts believe that if you have a sluggish thyroid, your body will channel available tyrosine to the gland to boost the production of thyroid hormone. When this happens, tyrosine may not be sufficiently available for the production of norepinephrine in the brain, which maintains a good mental outlook. As a result, depression may occur.

Dietary Guidelines for Low Thyroid Function

Avoid white sugar, white flour, red meat, milk, cheese, eggs and junk foods. Don't smoke or drink caffeine and alcohol. Keep in mind that thyroid medications such as Synthroid can help to correct the disorder, but they can also lead to osteoporosis. It is also true that if you can boost levels of circulating thyroid hormone, you may eliminate the need for antidepressant drugs altogether.

Interestingly, an unorthodox and relatively new treatment designed to stimulate the thyroid gland in people who are depressed is sleep deprivation. We mentioned earlier that depression sometimes improves in people who sleep less. These people may have hypothyroidism. Apparently the periodic controlled absence of sleep helps to restore normal levels of TSH (thyroid stimulating hormone) in some individuals.

Statistics tell us that up to 20 percent of people suffering from depression have a sluggish thyroid. Carefully consider the symptoms of hypothyroidism and insist that you doctor do the necessary tests to either rule out or confirm the disorder. For more information on the connection between the thyroid gland and depression see *Hypothyroidism, The Unsuspected Illness,* by Broda Barnes, M.D.

Supplement Game Plan for Dysfunctional Thyroid (Use with Core Protocol)

KELP
Typical dosage: Take as directed on product label. Kelp contains many trace elements. The most prominent and beneficial for thyroid function is iodine. Iodine is essential to the thyroid gland and the production of thyroid hormones. Iodine deficiency is known to produce obesity, goiters, dry skin and hair, and a reduced basal metabolic rate. Iodine can also protect the thyroid gland from radiation toxicity.

SIBERIAN GINSENG
Typical dosage: 100 to 200 mg daily of a product containing a minimum of one percent eleutheroside E. Siberian ginseng has a positive influence on the thyroid gland. It protects the gland from enlargement induced with thyroidin and atrophy induced by methylthiouracil. It also protects against radiation exposure.

ESSENTIAL FATTY ACIDS
Typical dosage: Use flaxseed and fish oil supplements and take them with your vitamin E supplement. Keep supplements refrigerated. These compounds are vital for glandular health and inhibit the types of inflammatory responses typically seen in autoimmune diseases like thyroid dysfunction. Take as directed on product labels.

DESICCATED THYROID
Typical dosage: Take as directed on product label. This natural supplement may help with mild forms of hypothyroidism and may also be supported by the addition of zinc and iodine.

Yeast Infections and Depression

More than fifty years ago, doctors began to strongly identify the yeast *Candida albicans* as a frequent cause of vaginal, mouth, throat and gastrointestinal tract infections. Orian Truss, M.D., of Birmingham was one of the first doctors to recognize that chronic yeast infections could cause mood disorders. For over twenty years, he has studied the correlation between yeast infections and a variety of complaints, including depression. His conclusion is that yeast infections affect their victims both physically and psychologically.

Several theories attempt to explain this connection, although at this writing none are really conclusive. Most experts believe that the presence of yeast disturbs the normal balance of intestinal flora (friendly bacteria), which can inadvertently affect mood. One other possibility is that the presence of a yeast infection reduces the ability of the liver to clear the bloodstream of toxic waste that impacts the brain.

Most medical doctors and scientists are skeptical of the link between yeast infections and depression. Getting the scientific data to conclusively support this relationship may take years to secure. In the meantime, observations like those of Dr. Truss should not be ignored. Some observant doctors have discovered that yeast and other fungal infections commonly accompany depression.

A DEFINITION OF YEAST INFECTION

Yeast infections are a generally misunderstood condition. A generalized yeast infection is a very serious condition and only occurs when the immune system is profoundly weakened; however, this infection is not the type of yeast infection I am referring to. Yeast lives within all of our systems, and when the biochemistry of those systems is healthy, the yeast causes us few problems. But many people experience a sensitivity to yeast that has grown on specific mucous membranes of the body, where the climate is moist and favorable. The vagina and the gastrointestinal tract are both susceptible to yeast infections. A yeast infection occurs when the del-

Candida's Ill-Effects

The fact that candida secretes an identifiable toxin is thought to be the most plausible reason for its effect on the nervous system. Some of these symptoms include fatigue, irritability, confusion, mood swings, headaches and depression. Repeated exposure to candida overgrowth (called *candidiasis*) and its resulting toxins is what some health experts believe causes yeast syndrome, which affects a variety of body systems, including the mood-controlling centers of the brain.

icate balance of microorganisms is disrupted. As a result, the yeast can rapidly multiply.

WHAT CAUSES YEAST TO OVERGROW?

The climate of the vagina is perfect for yeast proliferation. Men usually develop the infection somewhere in the digestive system, and in children it can show up in certain diaper rashes, thrush and ear infections.

How does one get a yeast infection? Taking antibiotics can create a favorable environment for this fungus by causing the type of imbalance we've just talked about. Antibiotics not only kill harmful bacteria, they do away with the friendly bacteria we need to maintain the proper ratio of microorganisms. For this reason, if you have to take antibiotics, make sure to take lactobacillus acidophilus to replace lost bacteria.

High blood sugar can also predispose the body to a yeast infection. Yeast infections are commonly seen in people with diabetes. The body changes associated with taking birth control pills and steroids can also affect the internal climate of areas prone to infection. Consuming white sugar, breads that are high in yeast, and drinking alcohol can promote yeast infections in some individuals.

In fact, a study of 100 women published in an issue of the

Symptoms of Chronic Yeast Infection (Candidiasis)

- acne
- bloating
- cramps
- craving for sweets
- depression
- diarrhea and/or constipation
- eczema
- excessive perspiration
- food intolerance
- gas
- headaches
- hives
- loss of sexual desire
- mood swings

- nail infections
- psoriasis
- PMS
- recurring vaginal or bladder infections
- vaginal discharge
- vaginal itching and burning
- water retention

(For Men)
- impotence
- genital rashes
- prostatitis
- recurring anal itching

If you suspect you might suffer from chronic yeast infections, you need to see a doctor. In recent years, it seemed as if every ailment was being attributed to yeast. Understandably, these unsubstantiated links were quickly scoffed at by most physicians. Despite the lack of credibility that accompanied such claims, physicians are beginning to realize that yeast infections are much more prevalent than previously thought, and that they can cause a myriad of other disorders. Be aware that candida is often missed by medical practitioners although a blood test for candidiasis is available from several accredited laboratories. This test detects the presence of candida antibodies in the bloodstream.

Journal of Reproductive Medicine found that the intake of sugar, dairy products and artificial sweeteners had a positive correlation with the incidence of *Candida vulvovaginitis*. After being placed on a diet that eliminated these substances, more than 90 percent of these women were free from yeast infections for over a year. Be aware also that the internal environment of the vagina can reflect the condition and health of the entire body.

YEAST AND THE MIND

Once you've had a yeast infection, you may find that they have a tendency to recur, and once a yeast infection has proliferated, it can create a chemical imbalance in the body that can affect the way amino acids are used. By now, we should be well aware of the fact that amino acids are crucial precursor compounds for the neuro-transmitter chemicals that keep our moods elevated. In fact, the body systems that are most affected by a chronic yeast infection are the brain and the female endocrine system.

It is the brain connection that I am most interested in. Someone suffering from a chronic yeast infection may have trouble concentrating or feel lethargic, irritable or depressed. The symptoms vary with each person. Another little-recognized consequence of yeast infections is that they can make you more sensitive to colds and environmental allergens such as weeds, grasses and pollen, which can also result in depression. Some doctors have found that when symptoms of a yeast infection cleared up, sensitivities to food and other potential allergens also improved.

Dietary Guidelines for Preventing and Treating Yeast Infections

Eliminate white sugar, white flour, quick-cooking grains and yeast breads. Avoid yeast, mold and fungus foods such as alcoholic beverages, citrus fruits, bakery products, aged cheese, vinegar, truffles, rich dairy foods, chocolate and caffeine. If you have decided to take Nystatin, which is commonly prescribed by doctors to kill a yeast infection, make sure you take lactobacillus acidophilus to replace the friendly bacteria that are destroyed. Eat plenty of live culture, low-fat yogurt. Increase your consumption of raw fresh fruits and vegetables and use oat, millet or rye instead of wheat. Keep your carbohydrate intake low until the infection is controlled. Also, using artificial sweeteners can increase the likelihood of yeast infections. Eat soy-based foods like tofu for natural estrogenic action.

Supplement Game Plan for Yeast Infections (Use with Core Protocol)

ACIDOPHILUS LIQUID OR CAPSULES
Typical dosage: These supplements replenish the friendly bacteria in the vagina needed to fight infection. The lactobacillus variety has been found to be the most effective. Take as directed on product label and look for products containing lactobacillus and check the expiration date. You should be getting up to two billion live organisms daily. You can also dissolve powdered acidophilus into sterile water and use as a vaginal douche.

GARLIC
Typical dosage: Look for a product that will supply you with a day's dosage of a minimum of 10 mg of alliin or 4,000 mcg of allicin. The compounds in garlic have proven antifungal properties that have been shown to be effective against some antibiotic-resistant organisms.

VITAMIN A AND BETA CAROTENE
Typical dosage: Up to 25,000 IU of vitamin A daily for two weeks, then reduce to 10,000 IU daily. If you are pregnant, do not exceed 10,000 IU daily. Vitamin A is necessary to maintain the health of the vaginal mucosa and to boost the immune system.

ZINC PICOLINATE
Typical dosage: Take 45 to 60 mg daily. Some studies have shown zinc to be toxic to vaginal yeast infections. A lack of zinc can also weaken the immune system, which can predispose one to infection. Topical zinc ointments can also be used for itching.

ECHINACEA

Typical dosage: Take 300 mg daily. Echinacea helps to boost white cell count for fighting infections.

TRANSFER FACTOR

Typical dosage: This molecule, isolated from bovine colostrum, helps to raise immune response by transferring immune memory from cows. Look for a patented product that contains pure transfer factor and use as directed on product label.

GOLDENSEAL ROOT

Typical dosage: Take 300 to 500 mg daily of a product containing an 8 percent alkaloid content. Goldenseal root has a long history of use for vaginitis because it creates stronger cross-links between the mucosal proteins of the vagina, making it much more difficult to disrupt the protective lining.

Note: Avoid taking iron supplements while the infection is active. Iron can feed certain bacteria. Also, do not use any B vitamins that are yeast based.

Low Cholesterol Levels and Depression

Surprising new evidence shows that although high cholesterol levels are not good, excessively low levels of cholesterol can also pose health threats—especially when it comes to state of mind. Psychiatric researchers at Duke University Medical Center found higher rates of depression and anxiety among young women with very low cholesterol, compared with women who had normal levels or higher. It may seem somewhat far-fetched, but it seems that makeup of our blood fats can impact our mood.

I have no doubt that many young women with extremely low cholesterol levels are eating diets that are virtually fat-free to maintain or lose weight. Fat phobias can result in dangerously low blood cholesterol levels that wreak havoc with our health. The link between low cholesterol and depression was also discovered in elderly men. Another study found higher suicide rates among men with very low cholesterol levels.

WHAT DOES CHOLESTEROL HAVE TO DO WITH DEPRESSION?

Cholesterol provides special building blocks for all body cells. If a cell lacks cholesterol, its structure can be impaired. In other words, cells can lose some of their strength and integrity if they are cholesterol deficient. In the brain, cells weakened by missing cholesterol components may be less receptive to mood-controlling chemicals like serotonin. The altered cell shape may not permit brain chemicals to fit properly in designated receptors, and the desired cellular effect is lost. While its mechanisms remain a bit of a mystery, the cholesterol link to mood once again underscores how important it is to keep all of our body systems in balance. Extremes of any kind can disrupt the delicate biochemical balance of the brain, and depression can result from some of the most unlikely circumstances.

Fibromyalgia, Pain and Mood

Considered one of today's mystery diseases, fibromyalgia is becoming an all too common disorder. Victims of this disorder (mainly women) are often unaware that they are suffering from a specific ailment. Fibromyalgia belongs to a family of disorders that are characterized by an overreaction to what is considered normal stimulus. Some of these are insomnia, irritable bowel syndrome and migraine headaches. Not too long ago, fibromyalgia was thought to be psychosomatic, which was particularly troubling to its victims. Since then, this theory fortunately has been discarded.

In fact, fibromyalgia is another in a long line of disorders considered by-products of western lifestyles rarely seen in underdeveloped countries. It has also been linked to emotional trauma or depression, and is characterized by muscular aches that affect common points of the body and cause burning, stiffness and chronic aching. It is usually accompanied by sleep disorders like an inability to fall into deep or restful sleep (where tissue healing and cell regeneration take place). Because of sleep disturbances, fatigue is often the result of the fibromyalgia cycle.

SUBSTANCE P, FIBROMYALGIA AND THE BRAIN

Recent scientific tests have found that people with fibromyalgia suffer from decreased cerebral blood flow and have higher levels of substance P in their system. (Remember that substance P is a chemical involved in pain transmission in the nervous system. It is also thought to play a role in mood disorders.) Clinical studies have found that blocking the action of substance P in some depressed people resulted in a dramatic improvement of mood. Can you see a possible connection here?

Dr. I. Jon Russell, Professor of Medicine and Clinical Immunology at the University of Texas Health Science Center at San Antonio, believes that substance P levels are abnormally elevated in the spinal fluid of people with fibromyalgia. He also discovered that people with fibromyalgia had a much lower pain threshold and that they had more trouble with anxiety and depression. In light of other studies which report that people with fibromyalgia also suffer from decreased blood flow to the brain, he believes that there is a relationship between the substance P level and this impaired blood flow.

ESTROGEN, SLEEP AND FIBROMYALGIA

Since women are the primary targets of fibromyalgia, some experts suggest a possible estrogen link to the disease. Sleeping disorders have also been linked to this disease, and some experts believe that fibromyalgia may reflect the biological havoc our bodies experience if we do not sleep properly. The chronic pain, the disturbed sleep, the fatigue and the depression that accompany this disease are thought to be the result of disturbances in biological rhythms.

Fibromyalgia is often preceded by a time of prolonged stress. Furthermore, SAMe, 5-HTP and essential fatty acids—all considered natural treatments for fibromyalgia—are also key compounds found in the core protocol for treating depression. This overlap is not a coincidence.

Supplement Game Plan for Fibromyalgia (Use with Core Protocol)

MALIC ACID
Typical dosage: Take 300 mg three times daily with magnesium supplement. This compound takes part in cell metabolic processes that help muscles to use glucose properly. This compound, a part of the Krebs cycle in the body, is thought to reduce the severity of symptoms associated with fibromyalgia, especially when combined with magnesium.

MAGNESIUM
Note: This can replace the recommendation for magnesium listed in the Core Protocol.
Typical dosage: Take 800 mg of magnesium daily. Use magnesium citrate, malate, fumarate, aspartate or succinate. This mineral works to support muscle cell function and has a synergistic action when combined with malic acid. Tests have found that magnesium stores may be depleted in women with fibromyalgia. Supplementation in test cases has resulted in significant improvement.

MANGANESE
Typical dosage: Take as directed or use SOD (superoxide dismutase), which is rich in manganese. Like magnesium, tests suggest that anyone suffering from a disease that causes chronic inflammation or pain may be suffering from a manganese deficiency.

Note: 5-HTP and St. John's wort have been used to treat fibromyalgia and are suggested in the core protocol for depression. If you have fibromyalgia, make sure to include these along with the other suggested supplements listed above.

CHAPTER 14

Depression: A Trigger of Disease

Discovery consists in seeing what everybody else has seen and thinking what nobody else has thought.

ALBERT SZENT-GYORGI

A CENTURY AGO, Dr. Henry Maudsley said, "The sorrow that has no vent in tears may make other organs weep." Henry aptly expresses what natural health practitioners have advocated for centuries—if we don't learn how to manage our emotional stresses, our biological selves will suffer. Up until now, this book has mainly discussed physical ailments as possible causes for depression, but the reverse is also true. Being depressed in and of itself can be a powerful catalyst for disease. New findings support the idea that the human body breaks down when subjected to prolonged periods of stress or sadness. What we often don't realize is how direct the biological effect of a low mood can be on seemingly unrelated things like blood sugar and heart health.

Keep in mind that 15–20 percent of people who have heart attacks also experience depression, as do 15 to 20 percent of people with diabetes according to the American Diabetes Association. And 25 percent of those with major depression also have a substance abuse problem. So, the question is, which comes first, the depression or the disease? More and more scientific data supports the idea that being down in the dumps can make you physically sick—and may even kill you. Solving the depression puzzle is not just about feeling happier or developing the skills it takes to understand illness and the body, it is essential for good health. This chapter will show you some of the ways that mood disorders can undermine your health and will hopefully convince you to take the necessary steps to problem-solve your own depression.

Feeling Glum Can Literally Break Your Heart

Research out of Columbia University reports that depression actually increases the likelihood of heart disease fatalities. Thousands of people were followed for over ten years, and in 1993, it was concluded that even after taking into account the effect of smoking, depression substantially increased the risk of sudden death from heart disease. The study also found that healthy people who become depressed are more likely than their counterparts who have no depression to develop heart disease approximately ten years after the depressive episode.

These statistics are startling and place your chances of having a heart attack somewhere between 50 and 100 percent more likely if you're forty-five, healthy and suffer from clinical depression. In other words, depression can make you over three times more likely to die from a heart attack.

Believe it or not, scientists now think that depression makes our blood platelets stickier, which in turn raises our risk of developing a blood clot. If such a clot breaks loose, it can impact the heart or decrease blood circulation to heart muscle. Researchers at Emory University in Atlanta have found that the platelets of depressed people are hypersensitive to certain body signals, which make them clump when they should remain fluid and flowing. These clumps can snag themselves on artery cracks or cholesterol deposits and eventually break away causing a heart attack. They can also build up to the point where blood supply to the heart is choked off.

Heart Rhythms, Blood Pressure and Depression

Not only does depression occur in up to half of those who have had heart attacks, some statistics even suggest that the risk of heart disease is three times higher in men who experienced periods of depression in their lives. Depressed men are more likely to develop coronary artery disease—a Johns Hopkins study reported that men with clinical depression are more than twice as likely to develop coronary artery disease (CAD) as their nondepressed counterparts.

In addition to the platelet connection, some researchers think that depression may cause potentially fatal changes in heart rhythms in people who are recovering from heart attacks. Other studies have suggested that depression also impairs the mechanisms that control our blood pressure. This particular problem can be counteracted by exercise, and experts suggest that depressed heart attack patients exercise as part of their recovery. Exercise not only helps to stabilize the electrical system of the heart, but also elevates brain chemicals that boost mood. The function that normally keeps our blood pressure at normal readings is called baroreflex control, and it seems to be abnormally low in people who have trouble with depression.

Depression Can Worsen Diabetes

The effect of depression on the heart is also a major concern for diabetics, who are at increased risk for heart disease. Diabetics with depression may also have a harder time controlling their blood sugar levels than emotionally healthy diabetics. According to a report, published in the October 1999 issue of the *Journal of Applied Psychophysiology & Biofeedback,* people with insulin-dependent diabetes who fight depression are the least likely to successfully lower their blood sugar levels. These findings have been so impressive that the American Diabetes Association suggests that a diabetic should target his or her depression first in order to effectively manage their blood sugar.

How feeling gloomy impacts blood sugar remains somewhat of a mystery. Some experts believe that depression may change levels of the adrenal hormone called cortisol, which can increase insulin resistance. Raising cortisol can also raise your risk of future heart disease as well.

It has long been known that people with diabetes are more susceptible to depression than the general population. Because the number one concern of diabetics is getting their blood sugar under control, their depression often goes unaddressed. As a result, these diabetics often lack the initiative to use exercise and good nutrition to control their diabetes. Depressed diabetics are also more prone to complications of diabetes such as heart disease, nerve damage and blindness. If you or someone you care about is diabetic and depressed, use the supplement core protocol to get their depression under control while addressing their blood glucose levels.

Prolonged Depression Causes Bone Loss

In addition to blood sugar links, depression can also affect bone mass and raise a women's risk of developing osteoporosis. In fact, new research has linked emotional stressors such as loneliness and depression to an increased risk of hip fractures in women over fifty. Not only does depression increase lack of concentration in some women that raises their risk of falls and accidents, researchers have also found that depression causes an increase in cortisol, which has been linked to bone loss (as well as insulin resistance and heart disease). High levels of circulating cortisol can rob the bones of the calcium they need to stay strong and flexible. Simply stated, depression accelerates changes in bone mass that lead to osteoporosis.

A recent article in the *New England Journal of Medicine* reported that the lifetime risk of fractures related to depression is substantial. Researchers at the National Institutes of Health found that depressed premenopausal women can develop bones as porous as the bones of postmenopausal women, and calcium-leaching persisted despite treatment with antidepressant drugs. Researchers reported that bone mineral density was, on average, 6 percent lower in the spines of twenty-four depressed women than among twenty-four test subjects in the control group. And in the hip bone, bone mineral density was 10 to 14 percent lower in the depressed subjects.

Depression Can Increase the Risk of Stroke

Studies have also uncovered an unlikely connection between depression and silent stroke—a brain condition that can lead to a stroke. A silent stroke occurs when small blood vessels in the brain rupture or become blocked. These strokes can go undetected because they don't produce the normal warning signs of stroke—dizziness, headache, etc. As time passes, these smaller blood vessels become unable to provide blood or oxygen to the brain and cells die off causing memory, concentration and motor-skill problems. Depression seems to aggravate silent strokes.

In a study published the *Journal of the American Heart Association,* researchers recommended that individuals who develop depression after age fifty be evaluated for stroke. If you have had problems with depression, some doctors believe that you could already have some of these abnormal vessels. They also strongly advise getting a handle on your depression to prevent further damage. Ironically, depression can also be a result of a silent stroke. Both depression and stroke are typically seen in the elderly, and as we talked about earlier, geriatric depression often goes untreated or is actually made worse by a whole host of drug interactions.

Depression May Be a Marker
for Alzheimer's Disease

New information also tells us that when an older person becomes depressed, it could be an early warning sign of Alzheimer's disease. A Swedish study tracked 222 persons age seventy-four and older for three years and found that the thirty-four people who developed Alzheimer's disease had many more symptoms of depression from the start of the study than those who did not develop the disease. Doctors should test a depressed older person's blood for folate and vitamin B12 levels, since deficiencies in both nutrients can cause malnutrition and lead to depression. Discovering Alzheimer's disease in its early stages can make treatment options more effective. Using *Ginkgo biloba*, for example, is much more effective in cases where the disease has not progressed.

Depression Can Weaken Your Immune System

Furthermore, a study published in a 1999 issue of *Psychosomatic Medicine* focusing on depressed women reported that depression actually lowers the number of natural killer cells produced by the immune system. These cells aggressively attack disease-carrying organisms, so when their count goes down, our susceptibility to sickness goes up. Even mild depression weakens the immune system, so the link between state of mind and our ability to fight disease is a profound one.

Dr. Marvin Stein of the Mt. Sinai School of Medicine at the City University of New York and his colleagues studied a group of widowers soon after they lost their wives and found a decrease in T and B cell activity of their immune systems. B and T cells kill microscopic disease-causing invaders. This may also help to explain why disorders like chronic fatigue syndrome, which is caused by the Epstein-Barr virus, is associated with depression.

Similar testing has shown that depressed people have significantly poorer DNA or genetic repair of their cells. Doctors at Ohio State University discovered that the cells of people who suffered from mood disorders regenerated at a slower rate when exposed to radiation. These findings suggest that emotional stress may contribute to the incidence of cancer by causing abnormal cell development or by weakening the bodies defense system against carcinogen exposure.

Unquestionably, there is a relationship between the severity of depression and suppression of the immune system. Doctors have also found that when depression subsides, T and B cell production increases. This particular phenomenon is not restricted to human beings alone.

Studies done with dogs showed similar results. A dog that was used to being loved and affectionately petted was left completely alone for an extended period of time. Although he was given plenty of nutritious food and an ample water supply, he was denied any physical contact. At periodic intervals, his bone marrow was checked for changes. After a couple of weeks, the dog acted depressed and changes in his white and red blood cell count occurred. In essence, his immune system was compromised—due to a simple lack of love and attention.

Whereas tests done at George Washington University on cancer patients found that those who engaged in regular relaxation exercises and used creative imagery to foster feelings of well-being and health experienced positive changes in their immune systems. The production of antibodies, lymphocytes and interleukin-2 messengers increased in proportion to their practice of stress-relieving exercise and creative mental imagery.

A Final Word

The message is clear. If we get depressed, whatever the reason, our ability to fight disease is inhibited and our health may be compromised. And as we have seen throughout the book, physical ailments can make the mind more prone to depression. Clearly, the connection between the body and the mind is so intrinsic to our health that illness in either can create a feedback loop that leads to illness in the other. Likewise, a healthy mind reinforces a healthy body and the reverse. For this reason, it's important to value both our physical and mental health. The human body and spirit thrive when their health is supported. Understanding this fact is essential to successfully deciphering the puzzle we call depression.

CHAPTER 15

Weight and Mood: The Chicken or the Egg?

A drop in mood can make you turn to food.
UNKNOWN

FOR MANY OF us, eating is how we attempt to pull ourselves out of the doldrums. For instance, as discussed earlier in the book, if you suffer from seasonal affective disorder (SAD), you may eat more than usual and put on weight. One of the symptoms of depression is weight change—either loss or gain, and because of this connection, we often connect eating with stress and depression. Therefore, this chapter will focus on the relationship between food and mood and provide compelling evidence that mood, appetite and weight are closely linked.

First, however, we need to dispel some common myths about weight and depression. Contrary to popular belief, depression does not necessarily cause us to gain weight, and depression is not more prevalent among people who are overweight. In fact, many people who are clinically depressed lose their appetite and desire to eat, and typically lose weight. In other words, there is no direct causal link between obesity and depression—one does not necessarily predispose someone to the other.

Nevertheless, with those biases and misconceptions aside, individuals who are obese (especially women) frequently fall into depressed mind-sets due to a number of factors, even though they are not necessarily more likely to be depressed than slimmer individuals. So what exactly is the connection between weight and depression?

Naturally, when we talk about individuals who are suffering with both obesity and depression, we face the old chicken and the egg dilemma. Do overeating, inactivity and weight gain lead to depression, or does depression cause overeating, inactivity and weight gain? This chapter will discuss another piece of the food-mood connection and the detrimental ways many individuals respond to it. I will also discuss natural solutions for depression influenced by these factors.

Obesity as a Result of Emotional Stress

For decades, experts believed that many people with weight problems overindulged in food as a reaction to certain forms of stress. In this theory, stress leads to overeating and weight gain, which results in depression, further stress and overeating. However, because current studies have found that obese people don't have a higher incidence of depression than other people, scientists are now revisiting that theory. It is true, however, that many of us eat when we are anxious or worried—a fact that has its roots in brain chemistry and appetite stimulation. And while data may tell us that overweight individuals are no more sad that we are, no one will contest the fact that being overweight is looked down on by our society and generates/reinforces negative thoughts and self-images.

Just to give you an idea of how devastating obesity can be, a survey by Rand and McGregor reported that 47 percent of patients who lost weight following surgery would rather become deaf, blind or diabetic than regain the weight they lost. Why? Because obese people typically face family, friends and employers who believe they are lazy, lack ambition and have lower IQs. Social rejection and discrimination in the workplace certainly contribute to low self-esteem and mood slumps. Nevertheless, just because emotional stressors like these can contribute to depression does not mean that they are the sole cause of depression.

Obesity and Depression

Most of us assume that overweight people become depressed because of society's distaste for fatness, which encourages self-rejection. And in fact, women—much more than men—can become very unhappy about their weight and commonly feel depressed, undesirable and rejected. Our body image profoundly impacts our emotional landscape, and poor body image is linked to depression and low self-esteem (just ask any adolescent girl). There is no question that societal rejection and judgement play a part in depression.

Furthermore, many obese people are frequently disappointed in the attention and care they receive when they go to their doctors for help. What is particularly troubling is the fact that many of them feel that their doctors look down upon them as people. In her book, *The Carbohydrate Addict's Lifespan Program,* Dr. Rachel Heller relates her physician's reaction to her obesity. After seeing her heavy body, which weighed over 300 pounds, his comments to her as her healer and confidant were, "You are fat for one reason and one reason only. You eat like a pig. You look like a pig because you eat like a pig, and you will continue to look like a pig until you stop eating like a pig." She goes on to say that she did not overeat because she was lazy or self-indulgent. She was literally addicted to food. Much like an alcoholic, she could not stop herself from eating, and it was literally killing her. Instead of helping her get to the real cause of her appetite and weight problems, her doctor belittled her and gave her a food exchange diet to follow.

Heller's book provides another look at the food-mood connection. As mentioned earlier in this chapter, weight gain and mood slumps are only two pieces in the puzzle; however, there is another puzzle piece that is intrinsically connected to both depression and obesity—carbohydrate metabolism disorder.

Carbohydrate Binging: The Missing Piece

Neurochemical research backs up Dr. Rachel Heller's idea that a physical reason underpinned her obesity. I talked about this idea earlier when I first cited the Wurtman study, which found that people who crave and eat excess carbohydrates may be more prone to depression and obesity. Typically, carbohydrate addicts begin to overeat in the late afternoon and evening when they continually consume an array of carbohydrate snack foods. It is this sustained snacking that dramatically increases their caloric intake for the day, resulting in weight gain.

We now know that as many as two-thirds of all obese people are carbohydrate cravers, suggesting that they overeat, not because they are gluttons, but because they suffer from a carbohydrate metabolism disorder. What is carbohydrate metabolism disorder? As I discussed in Chapter 6, people who binge on carbohydrates may be suffering from a malfunction in the area of the brain that tells them to stop eating. In these cases, the brain fails to respond the way it should when carbohydrates are eaten, which explains why one or two cookies is never enough. In fact, such binging can become automatic—sufferers do not even realize how much they are eating.

In keeping with the Wurtman study findings, other tests have found that overweight carbohydrate cravers are frequently depressed and admit that their eating is motivated by a strange kind of insatiable hunger. They eat to find feelings of comfort and well-being that certain foods seem to provide. How do these foods promote happiness? They affect serotonin levels in the brain. It was this brain chemistry link (serotonin) that led to the creation of diet drugs like Redux and fenfluramine, which raise serotonin levels in the brain and promote positive feelings. The pills were very effective for thousands of people but came with dangerous side effects.

Therefore, the problem of carbohydrate metabolism disorder is twofold. Not only do sufferers crave carbohydrates to fight off stress, depression and fatigue, they also binge on carbohydrates because their brains do not signal them to stop eating. Both factors lead to weight gain and further mood disorders. The excessive carbohydrates they crave interfere with natural mood enhancement and lead to further addiction and depression. So while obesity in and of itself does not cause depression and depression is not necessarily the cause of weight gain, being addicted to carbohydrates can make one prone to both weight gain and depression. And each factor reinforces the others.

Why some people become carbohydrate dependent and some do not has a lot to do with the hormone insulin. Insulin regulates the metabolism of carbohydrates—taking glucose (from the carbohydrates) out of the blood and depositing it in the cells for energy. Insulin also signals when we need glucose. Disruptions in this process can not only lead to diabetes and hypoglycemia, they can also interfere with energy levels, weight and of course, mood (since sugar directly affects brain chemistry). The more I learn about insulin, the more convinced I am that learning to control its secretion is one of the healthiest things we can do. I know that I have a problem with sugars and starches, and insulin reactions certainly influence my moods, productivity and weight. I saw the same pattern in my father and grandmother and so I have to believe that a genetic component is at work here.

The Genetic Link to Eating Disorders and Depression

Genes may also play a role in the development of eating disorders accompanied by depression. Scientists at the Virginia Institute for Psychiatric and Behavioral Genetics recently conducted a study supporting the idea that anorexia and depression share common risk factors. In other words, if you are prone to one, you may be prone to the other. The study concluded that heredity plays a major role in both conditions and they often appear simultaneously. Using over 2,000 female twin volunteers, the study found that genetics can have a very strong influence is the development of anorexia. Once again, this study suggests that the link between the food, mood and brain structure is a profound one. The brain chemistry behind anorexia and depression also impacts binge eaters and girls with bulimia.

Stress, Sugar and Weight Gain

Genes linked to obesity are also connected to depression and anxiety in some people. This discovery brings home the idea that behavior, metabolism, appetite and mood are connected. For many overweight individuals, therefore, the focus should be on getting healthy rather than on weight loss alone. The best thing in managing both depression and weight is to reduce high stress levels.

I've heard several women say that they seem to gain weight more easily when they are under periods of high stress. Naturally, most of us would assume that nervous eating associated with stress is what puts on pounds, but there is much more to stress-induced weight than caloric intake alone.

Scientists at the University of Virginia have studied the relationship between stress and glucose. Apparently, during times of stress, glucose is released as a result of an increase in the hormone epinephrine (adrenaline). Excess blood glucose stimulates LPL (lipoprotein lipase) or what has been called the "fat enzyme," resulting in the storage of excess body fat.

To make matters worse, during periods of stress, the body craves high-fat, high-glycemic foods. Because Americans are especially prone to stress-related maladies, learning how to prevent stress-induced weight is vital. Moreover, the fact that stress makes it easier to pack on the pounds may be a contributing factor to the never-ending obesity battle. One way to counteract this stress-motivated weight gain is to control our blood sugar and insulin levels.

Dieting and Eating Disorders

Paul Saltman, Ph.D., in the *California Nutrition Book,* says,

[F]ood is fun and sound nutrition need not diminish the pleasure. More than anything else, it's the nonsense of nutrition—the unreasonable food fears and unnecessary prohibitions that take the joy out of eating. Without an adequate amount and proper balance of nutrients, you are simply not going to live as long or as healthily, look as good, or work as hard as you are genetically programmed to do.

Unfortunately, in an attempt to attain the "perfect body" many of us have compromised our health in order to be thin. Dangerous diets and eating disorders such as bulimia can significantly contribute to depressive illness, especially among young women. Consistently going off and on diets, using diet pills, and binging and purging exact enormous physical and emotional tolls on our society. Often weight loss is bought at the expense of our health and happiness.

For years, psychiatrists assumed that the reason overweight people seemed more vulnerable to depressive illness centered around their dissatisfaction with how they looked. New research has found that the constant cycle of dieting frequently causes moods to plummet. The yo-yo syndrome of losing and gaining weight, in addition to the continual nutritional stress of dieting, directly impacts the mind. Combine this stress with possible carbohydrate metabolism disorder, and you have a recipe for disaster. Unfortunately, dieting is a way of life in our country.

Yes, I know what you're thinking—there's nothing like the "high" of feeling slender. Granted, it is a great feeling, but how you got there can spoil your euphoria. The results of unhealthy dieting can damage your health and disrupt your brain chemistry. Very low-calorie diets can cause serious depression. In addition to the risks of extreme caloric deprivation, the guilt and discouragement that result when hunger finally sabotages your diet plans only compound mood slumps.

The *Journal of Health and Social Behavior* reports that researchers asked over 2,000 men and women between the ages of eighteen and ninety to complete a standard checklist designed to detect symptoms of depression. The questionnaire also surveyed dietary and exercise habits, weight, height, etc. The study concluded that dieting was the leading cause of depression in overweight people. After looking at the data, the researchers strongly recommended that overweight individuals burn more calories rather than trying to eliminate them. Making exercise a regular part of one's lifestyle is the best alternative for overweight individuals. The study stated that "for mental health, the overweight would be best served by increasing their exercise levels rather than dieting, if they want to lose weight."

Dieting Can Deplete Serotonin

Why is exercise so much better for mental health than dieting? Starvation diets decrease supplies of norepinephrine, which can create mental lethargy and feelings of indifference. People who suffer from bulimia often have lower-than-normal levels of serotonin as well, and it's a well-known fact that bulimia is closely linked to depressive illness. The low serotonin levels of people with bulimia may also explain the uncontrollable carbohydrate binging that characterizes the disease. The fact that Prozac has met with some success in treating bulimia again underscores the profound link between food and mood.

This serotonin connection may also explain why dieting is so hard for most of us. If the type of diet we choose brings serotonin levels down, we may not be able to deal with how we feel. The classic symptoms of dieting—irritability, depression, moodiness and nervousness—may actually be caused by a serotonin deficiency, which may explain why a highly restrictive diet is usually followed by a carbohydrate-eating rampage. We may feel guilty, but our mood will certainly improve for a time. The Wurtman study we referred to in earlier sections has concluded that diets that are free of carbohydrates will ultimately fail because they are not "brain friendly."

If serotonin levels are so crucial to both depression and carbohydrate craving, amino acid and vitamin therapy, which are infinitely safer than diet pills or stimulants, may be extremely valuable in helping to control neurotransmitters levels. These therapies are discussed in more detail later in the chapter.

A NOTE ON DIET PILLS AND DEPRESSION

A study done at the University of San Francisco found that of 500 girls, nearly 50 percent of nine-year-olds and 80 percent of ten- and eleven-year-olds were dieting. The enormous number of girls who excessively diet and use over-the-counter appetite suppressants is cause for considerable concern, especially considering the effects of diet pills on the mental health of our young people.

Vivian Hanson Meechan, president of the National Association of Anorexia Nervosa and Associated Disorders, said, "Diet pills containing the drug phenylpropanolamine or PPA pose a very serious health risk to adolescents." PPA is commonly found in over-the-counter diet pills that claim to control hunger. She went on to disclose that at least one of every ten teenagers engages in dangerous eating practices, including starvation diets, binge eating, vomiting, abusing laxative and diuretics, and taking diet pills. PPA can cause nervousness, anxiety, severe mood swings, depression, high blood pressure and dizziness—just to name a few of its side effects. Frequently, teenage and college-age girls will live on diet pills, sacrificing their health for their looks.

Binge Eating and Mood

Pills are not the only response to restrictive diets. As mentioned earlier, binge eating can be another way to cope with them. This response to food is also linked to a carbohydrate metabolism disorder, and it is not a normal behavior. When hunger controls are impaired and brain chemicals aren't balanced, appetite can become a monster. Simply stated, binge eating involves a loss of control over how much food you eat.

This disorder affects 4 to 5 percent of obese individuals and is commonly seen among young bulimic women who frequently combine it with purging (vomiting). Binge eating is often the result of severely restrictive dieting, which prompts a person go on an eating tirade in order to restore brain chemicals, blood sugar and fats to proper levels. In fact, binge eating often becomes a type of antidepressant. The carbohydrates consumed by binge eaters serve to boost mood even while they undermine self-esteem. People with a carbohydrate metabolism disorder may eat a whole bag of potato chips in an attempt to raise their mood and energy level rather than to satisfy true hunger.

Keep in mind that binge eating not only depletes vital nutrients and chemicals that keep mood elevated, it also creates guilt and self-loathing. Anyone who has experienced binge eating with or without purging is very vulnerable to depression. Like anorexia, new studies tell us that bulimia and major depression have common genetic and environmental factors. And both restrictive dieting and binge eating only perpetuate the diet-depression cycle.

Binging, Hypoglycemia and Fat Storage

Another binge-eating trigger is low blood sugar or hypoglycemia. Hypoglycemia can cause uncontrollable eating binges of sugary or starchy foods—a fact that may explain why individuals with hypoglycemia tend to gain weight. In addition, hypoglycemia—like stress—causes the stimulation of lipoprotein lipase (LPL), the "fat enzyme." When insulin release is stimulated, so are the biochemical pathways that store fat.

Experts now believe that eating a food that consists of white sugar and dietary fat is even more prone to end up on the hips. Sucrose or table sugar has a specific effect on lipoprotein lipase. When sucrose teams up with dietary fat, LPL is stimulated, which prompts the release of triglycerides into the blood, resulting in more fat accumulation.

Unfortunately, the very foods we usually crave during a hypoglycemic episode are a combination of sucrose and fat—cookies, chips, doughnuts, cake, muffins, etc. Foods high in sugar stimulate LPL, causing the expansion of fat cells, which results in weight gain. Reducing our consumption of high-fat, high-glycemic foods can reverse this effect and keep us from binging.

Are You a Binge Eater?

Look over the following list of behaviors to see if you have a tendency to binge on food.

1. You eat very rapidly during a short amount of time, resulting in the consumption of large quantities of food.
2. You feel that you cannot control what, when and how much you eat.
3. You consistently eat very quickly.
4. You eat until you feel uncomfortably full and bloated.
5. You constantly eat small amounts of food even when you are not hungry.
6. You eat alone or secretly because you feel ashamed about how much you are consuming.
7. You experience self-depreciating thoughts, depression or guilt after having eaten too much.
8. You typically eat large amounts of food when you are tired, anxious, lonely, depressed or bored.

SOME OTHER FACTS ABOUT BINGE EATING

• Binge eating is a cause of marked distress.
• Binge eating occurs at least two days per week on average, and for over six months.
• True binge eating does not involve induced vomiting.

Keep in mind that if you are a binge eater, you may be suffering from the same type of chemical imbalance in the brain that causes depressive illness. See a doctor and consider changing your diet and using the core supplementation plan for treating depression, as well as other suggestions offered at the end of this chapter. Don't go on restrictive diets in order to compensate for your binging, and if you've become accustomed to vomiting after eating, see a doctor as soon as possible. Bulimia is a dangerous disease.

How to Avoid Dangerous Diets

Nothing sparks more interest than the latest weight-loss diet. Unfortunately, many of us plunge head-first into diet plans that promise miracle weight loss but actually do little more than deliver bad health. The following weight-loss strategies will only serve to ruin your health and possibly cut years off your life:

• binge eating and purging
• diet pills or other supplements that pose a health risk
• extreme exercising
• fad diets that advise eating in radical or restrictive ways
• nutrient-deficient diets
• restrictive dieting (less than 1000 calories a day)
• starvation routines or fasting

Remember that starving, binging and purging are all potentially dangerous behaviors that only serve to severely compromise one's physical and emotional health. If you engage in any of these behaviors, find a specialist who can help you balance your body systems. We've established the fact that people who are prone to eating disorders may also be prone to depression. If you are depressed, use the core protocol to treat depression and combine it with the suggested game plan for safe weight loss offered at the end of this chapter.

Can Antidepressant Drugs Cause Weight Gain?

I can't finish a discussion on weight and depression without discussing the effects of antidepressants on weight. I have heard countless women on Prozac say that they expected to lose weight while on the drug but just the opposite occurred. While Prozac is listed as an antidepressant drug that kills appetite, weight gain can still occur. Why? In some people, Prozac creates a feeling of extreme mellowness, which in some cases prompts a severe case of apathy. Some women on Prozac have commented that they just don't care about keeping their house clean, getting their bills paid on time, exercising every day or watching what they eat. Granted, this effect is not seen in everyone that takes the drug, but it does happen.

Data tells us that weight gain is frequently seen when antidepressant therapy is started, especially with tricyclic drugs. Interesting studies show that MAOIs and many antipsychotic drugs can cause weight gain. In fact, the weight can stay even when the drugs are stopped. Discontinuing drug treatment is usually not enough to stimulate weight loss, and a low-calorie diet is often recommended.

Depression Drugs that Affect Appetite and Weight Gain

DRUGS THAT MAY PROMOTE WEIGHT GAIN

Antidepressants	Antipsychotics
• amoxapine	• chlorpromazine
• amitriptyline	• haloperidol
• desipramine	• ioxapine
• doxepin	• mesoridazine
• imipramine	• perphenazine
• nortriptyline	• thioridazine
• phenelzine	• thiothixene
• tranylcypromine	• trifluoperazine
• trazodone	
• trimipramine	

DRUGS THAT MAY PROMOTE WEIGHT LOSS

• bupropion
• fluoxetine and other inhibitors of serotonin recapture
• molindone

Supplement Game Plan for Safe and Effective Weight Loss (Use with Core Protocol)

FIBER SUPPLEMENT

Typical dosage: Adding a fiber supplement to your diet can help reduce blood sugar, control appetite and promote feelings of fullness. Study after study supports its efficacy in promoting weight loss. Take in the morning and at night using products designed to mix in liquid. It is essential that you drink plenty of water.

GARCINIA CAMBOGIA (HCA)

Typical dosage: 500 mg three times daily with meals. This compound interferes with the conversion of carbohydrates to fat and is an excellent supplement to any weight loss program.

CARNITINE AND METHIONINE

Typical dosage: Helps to promote the creation of lean muscle mass while inhibiting hunger. Take as directed on an empty stomach with fruit juice.

The following compounds appear in the core protocol for depression but are also recommended for weight loss:

5-HTP (5-HYDROXYTRYPTOPHAN)

Note: This replaces the dosage recommendation for 5-HTP found in the Core Protocol.

Typical dosage: Use 50 to 100 mg three times daily. A twelve-week study in Rome administered oral 5-HTP to participants without any dietary restriction and weight loss averaged four pounds per week. The drug is a serotonin precursor and inhibits the desire to eat carbohydrates.

GTF CHROMIUM

Note: This replaces the dosage recommendation for GTF chromium found in the Core Protocol.

Typical dosage: Take 300 to 600 mg per day. This mineral increases the ability of body cells to utilize insulin, which plays a vital role in appetite control, thermogenesis, and the creation of muscle mass. Low levels of this nutrient have been discovered in obese individuals and supplementation has initiated weight loss.

OMEGA-6 AND OMEGA-3 FATTY ACIDS
Typical dosage: Take as directed using flaxseed, evening primrose and fish oil blends. Take a vitamin E supplement whenever you take fish oil. These compounds stimulate brown fat activity, where calories are burned. Individuals who have trouble losing weight repeatedly can benefit from this supplement.

L-TYROSINE
Note: This replaces the dosage recommendation for L-tyrosine found in the Core Protocol.
Typical dosage: Start with 500 mg three times daily, working to 1,000 mg. Tyrosine raises serotonin and other brain neurotransmitters to help discourage eating. Take on an empty stomach with fruit juice.

It's important to remember that if you are working with an overweight person and you neglect to address his or her depression, you may be encouraging potentially dangerous behavior in the form of drastic diets or eating disorders.

Additional Tips for Weight Loss

• Acupuncture stimulates certain meridian points that can help suppress the appetite, which can be beneficial for those wanting to lose weight.
• Avoid eating when you are anxious, bored or frustrated. Find something else to do when you feel inclined to eat under these circumstances, especially while reading or watching television. Sedentary lifestyles have been strongly linked to obesity. If you have to eat during these activities, munch on raw vegetables or nuts.

A Note on Weight Gain and Food Allergies

Once again, the notion that food allergies may play a role in obesity is worth investigating. Some very intriguing clinical studies have found that when people ate foods they were sensitive to, they gained weight, and when they eliminated these foods, they lost weight. The interesting thing about these studies is that caloric intake remained the same in both instances, suggesting that many more factors are involved in weight control than we may have assumed.

• Avoid fad diets. They not only make your body feel starved, but also lower your metabolism by slowing down your fat-burning processes.
• Avoid nibbling after the meal is over. Mothers are particularly susceptible to this. While they may eat sensibly during the meal, picking at leftovers while putting dishes away can significantly contribute to weight gain.
• Be patient. More permanent results will be obtained if weight loss is gradual. Remember that it takes time for the body to re-adjust to its new programmed weight.
• Don't chew gum. Chewing gum can activate the flow of gastric juices and make you feel like eating.
• Don't eat when you are depressed, lonely or angry.
• Don't use food as a reward.
• Drink at least eight glasses of water each day to avoid constipation.
• Eat only when you are truly hungry. Thirst is often mistaken for hunger. Drink when you feel the urge to eat, and if you are still hungry, then eat.
• Eating too fast or chewing improperly can also result in the consumption of more calories in less time. People who eat too fast can often become hungry again soon after eating. Eating a diet

that is high in fiber can automatically increase chewing time and slow the eating process. Also, listen to calm, soothing music while you eat and chew slowly.

- Exercise regularly. Exercise is considered by far the best method to control weight. Begin slowly by taking a ten-to-fifteen minute walk every three days, then walk every day, and then slowly increase your distance and your pace. Light exercise right after eating can help burn calories that have just been consumed.
- In order to lose weight, your body must use up more calories than are consumed. You must create an energy deficit. The rest of these suggestions may help to expedite the creation of that deficit.
- Join a support group that takes a sensible and healthful approach to losing weight. Be wary of diet organizations that are costly or limit you to their foods. Ediets at www.ediets.com is getting good reviews for its diet program and costs a mere ten dollars a month. Their diet profile and their newsletter are free.
- Keep all high-calorie foods on high shelves or on the back shelves of the refrigerator or don't buy them. Make low-calorie foods more easily accessible.
- Using diuretics or laxatives to induce weight loss is potentially hazardous to your health and results only in temporary weight loss.

CHAPTER 16

Drugs and Toxins that Contribute to Depression

Depression is often a side effect of drug usage, particularly of substances not often considered drugs, i.e. oral contraceptives, caffeine and cigarettes.

MICHAEL T. MURRAY, N.D.

WE ARE SURROUNDED by chemicals. We choose to take some of these chemicals into our bodies in the form of medications, while a whole host of other frightening chemicals remain hidden from our view. In this chapter we'll discuss the effect of medications, nicotine, caffeine, alcohol and environmental pollutants on our minds, since they may be significant pieces in your depression puzzle.

Clearly, using certain drugs can cause symptoms of depression in some people. If you can't figure out why you feel depressed, before you do anything else, look at the drugs you may be taking. These include both prescription and over-the-counter preparations. Depression can be a side effect of drug usage. Any time we take a drug, we may be disrupting the normal balance of monoamines in the brain that determine mood.

The first indication that depression might be caused by a biochemical imbalance in the brain came in the fifties when several patients who were being treated with resperine for hypertension became depressed. A similar scenario resulted with patients who were given iproniazid, an antituberculosis drug. How many other drugs that we take so trustingly cause our unexplained depression? Let's talk about one of the highest risk groups for drug-induced depression—the elderly.

Drugs and Geriatric Depression

An article written in the *Journal of the American Geriatric Society* stated: "Drugs, either prescribed by a physician or taken independently, often are responsible for the development of depression, the aggravation of a pre-existing depression or the production of depression-like symptoms such as sedation, apathy and lethargy." This article goes on to point out that many elderly people are not suffering from senility but from the depressive side effects of the handful of drugs they take every day.

In addition, new research published in the same journal reveals that depression, not senility or poor-fitting dentures, is the real cause of weight loss in most nursing home patients. Depression was found to be the true cause of weight loss in 37 percent of 156 nursing home residents who lost five pounds or more. The question we must ask is "how much of that depression was drug induced?" Geriatric doctors rarely address depression in the elderly, and most geriatric symptoms are shrugged off as part of the aging process. This belief is false. Depression is not normal, no matter how young or old you are.

Accutane May Cause Suicidal Tendencies

Recent reports on Accutane provide a classic example of how serious the side effects of some drugs can be. In 1998, the Food and Drug Administration advised consumers and doctors that the prescription, anti-acne drug Accutane (isotretinoin) had been linked to reports of depression, psychosis and even suicidal thoughts. Depression had been listed as a possible side effect of Accutane, but drug companies are now emphasizing the risk directly on Accutane labels. People who experienced this effect said that when they got off the drug, the depression subsided. If they resumed treatment, however, it came back. Unfortunately, many doctors neglect to warn their patients that the prescription they are so quick to scribble out may cause serious depression. For some people, Accutane can even be life threatening.

Steroids and Depression

Another example of drug-induced depression is found with steroid use. Specifically, using corticosteroids, which are prescribed for a variety of ailments, can cause depression—especially in young people. Physicians in Italy report that one five-year-old girl who was given cortisone for chronic hepatitis became increasingly depressed until she was totally uncommunicative and had uncontrollable crying spells. They traced her depressive state to the corticosteroid drug. If you must take steroid drugs, some research has suggested that supplementing the diet with vitamin C may help to counteract this particular side effect. Of course, steroid drugs come with a whole host of health risks and should be taken only if absolutely necessary.

Over-the-Counter and Prescription Antihistamines and Mood

Although Accutane and steroids may not be a concern for many people, certain over-the-counter antihistamine medications are taken in large amounts by the general population for common sinus problems and can also depress the nervous system. I've had some experience with this effect during allergy season. I noticed that when I took a twelve-hour cold cap, I would feel unusually low and pessimistic. As long as I took the medication, the depression persisted, and my moods continued to drop. The effect was so pronounced that friends and relatives became concerned about my attitude. Although I don't believe the package referred to this as a possible side effect, it surely was. Some products do state that their usage may depress the nervous system, but this is hardly an ade-

Table 1. Drugs that can contribute to depression.

Some Antihistamines
Antibiotics
- cycloserine (Seromycin)
- tetracyclines
- neomycin
- metronidazole (Flagyl)
- sulfonamides (Bactrim, Azo, Gantanol, Cotrim, Septra)
- gram-negative antibiotics

Anti-inflammatory Drugs
- Indocin
- Naprosyn

Antimalarials
- sulfadoxine
- pyrimethamine (Daraprim, Fansidar)

Arthritis/
Pain Relievers
- phenylbutazone (Azolid, Butazolidin)
- indomethacin (Indocin)
- piroxicam (Feldene)
- sulfasalazine (Azulfidine)
- aspirin
- phenacetin (A.P.C. w/ codeine)

Birth Control Drugs/
Synthetic Hormones
- estrogens
- progestins
- steroids

Chemotherapy
- vinblastine sulfate (Velban)
- Methotrexate
- procarbazine hydrochloride (Matulane)

Diet Pills
- amphetamines (Obetrol, Dexedrine, Desoxyn)
- benzphetamine (Didrex)
- diethylpropion hydrochloride (Tenuate, Tepanil)
- phenmetrazine hydrochloride (Preludin)
- mazindol (Sanorex, Mazanor)
- fenfluramine hydrochloride (Pondimin)
- phendimetrazine tartrate (Plegine, Melfiat, Bontril)
- phentermine (Ionamin, Fastin, Adipex-P)

Diuretics
- furosemide
- triamterene (Dyazide, Dyrenium)

Table 1 (cont.). Drugs that can contribute to depression.

Heart Medications
- digitalis (Digoxin, Lanoxin, Cedilanid, Crystodigin)
- procainamide (Pronestyl, Procan SR)

High Blood Pressure Medications
- hydralazine (Apresazide Apresoline)
- methyldopa (Aldomet, Aldoclor, Aldoril)
- clonidine hydrochloride (Catapres, Combipres)
- guanethidine (Ismelin, Esimil)
- propanolol hydrochloride (Inderal, Inderide)
- bethanidine
- reserpine (Chloroserpine, Regroton, Diupres, Diutensen-R, Hydropres, Serpasil, Unipres, Ser-AP-Es, Naquival, Metatensin, Hydromox, Hydro-Fluserpine)

Parkinson's Disease Medications
- amantadine hydrochloride (Symmetrel)

- levodopa (Larodopa, Sinemet CR)

Drugs for Psychosis
- phenothiazines (Compazine, Phenergan, Sparine, Stelazine, Temaril, Thorazine)
- haloperidol (Haldol)
- thioxanthene (Navane)

Seizure Medications
- succinimide (Celontin, Zarontin, Milontin)
- carbamazepine (Tegretol)
- mephenytoin (Mesantoin)

Sleeping Medications/ Tranquilizers
- Librium
- Valium
- barbiturates
- over-the-counter sleep aids

Other Drugs
- disulfiram (Antabuse)
- physostigmine (Antilirium)
- Tagamet
- choline (in large doses)
- lecithin (contains choline)
- cholestyramine

quate warning. In fact, for anyone who is already battling gloom, taking seemingly harmless antihistamines may turn their mild mood slump into severe depression.

Nicotine and Depression: A Vicious Cycle

In addition to prescription and over-the-counter drugs, various other pollutants can affect our mood. New studies report that people who are susceptible to depression also find it extremely difficult to stop smoking. Some experts believe that up to half of all smokers suffer from some degree of depression, and the overwhelming majority of these smokers fail when they try to quit. In light of these studies, some doctors are turning to antidepressant drugs like Prozac as a strategy for depressed smokers who want to stop smoking. In fact, a study conducted by the Department of Psychiatry at the University of California at San Francisco reported, "Depressed smokers appear to experience more withdrawal symptoms on quitting, are less likely to be successful at quitting, and are more likely to relapse."

What are the reasons for this phenomenon? Well, first of all, nicotine is closely linked to emotional state and removing it from the system can be particularly devastating, especially for people with mood disorders. Just to give you an idea of how powerfully tobacco can elevate mood, a recent study suggested using nicotine patches as a legitimate treatment for depression! Talk about a mixed up world.

In any case, when people who are prone to mood slumps try to cut down on cigarette usage, they become severely depressed. Hence, they light up again. However, although it may be one of the hardest thing you'll ever accomplish, the best thing you can do for yourself if you are a smoker who suffers with clinical depression is to kick the nicotine habit. Simply stated, if you are suffering from depression, stop smoking. If you're not suffering from depression, stop smoking.

Andrew Weil, M.D., tells us that smoking puts dangerous drugs into the brain more directly than would an intravenous injection.

Smoking affects mood through the action of carbon monoxide, which is toxic to brain cells. In addition, ingesting nicotine can significantly lower vitamin C levels and lead to a vitamin deficiency, and a lack of vitamin C not only leads to gum disease, it can also contribute to a number of neurotic symptoms, including depression.

To make matters worse, smoking stimulates the adrenal glands to secrete adrenaline and cortisol. Cortisol inhibits the uptake of tryptophan by brain cells, which results in lowered levels of serotonin. By now, we should be all too aware that decreased serotonin levels cause depression, and that excess cortisol is not good for our mood or our weight.

Nicotine can also potentiate the effect of caffeine and sugar on the system, two more mood disrupters. So, if you typically eat a Danish for breakfast and have a cigarette and a Coke on your break, you're setting the stage for conditions like depression. In fact, nicotine belongs to the same family of addictive substances as alcohol, caffeine and sugar. When we feel lousy, many of us grab a doughnut, pour ourselves a drink, or light one up, and although we may feel better initially, in the long term, we will feel worse. Like any drug, the effects of nicotine are only temporary, and if you smoke, your mood and energy levels will eventually drop. These drops only reinforce the whole destructive cycle and encourage further use of these destructive influences in order to cope.

The Caffeine Connection to Depression

Caffeine is the most widely used drug in our society. It is found in a number of foods, medications and beverages, and the average American consumes 150 to 225 mg of caffeine each day. We could write an entire book on negative biological effects of caffeine alone, which makes it a very significant piece in the complex puzzle of factors that contribute to the onset of depression.

Caffeine alters brain amine function, and the intake of caffeine has been positively correlated with the degree of mental illness in some psychiatric patients. In addition, caffeine becomes even more potent when combined with sugar—a particularly bad duo, and the two are often found and ingested together.

Not convinced? Consider the fact that heavy coffee drinkers consistently score higher on tests for depression and anxiety than control groups. Coffee contains from 29 to 176 mg of caffeine, cola drinks contain about 40 mg, and a chocolate bar approximately 25 mg. Even if you eliminate these substances from your diet, you need to watch for hidden sources of caffeine found in various medicines and appetite suppressants.

In fact, on average, an individual who consumes three cups of coffee, a chocolate candy bar, a cola drink and two headache pills can consume around 400 mg of caffeine in one day—an amount that is linked to severe mental and emotional disturbances. In fact, consuming 250 mg of caffeine has been linked to a number of disturbed behaviors.

Do you know how much caffeine you consume in a day? Our society is becoming so caffeine dependent that psychiatrists have coined a new phrase for the problem in their diagnostic manual—caffeinism. Not only has our obsession with caffeine made it the most widely used drug in the world, cola drinks are the most popular beverages in this country and are routinely consumed by children. However, the festive and fun cola commercials fail to tell us that caffeine is actually a strong and addicting drug.

CAFFEINE CREATES BRAIN CHAOS

How exactly does caffeine affect the way your brain and nervous system work? Caffeine initially stimulates the release of norepinephrine, which actually results in a temporary lift in mood; however, over time, brain amine supplies can become depleted. The results of excess caffeine consumption are insomnia, fatigue, anxiety, panic attacks, delirium and wild mood fluctuations.

In fact, a study published in *Life Science* magazine reported that caffeine causes neurons stimulated by serotonin to decrease the conversion of tryptophan to the compound that will eventually become serotonin. This effect can result in a depressive episode. Caffeine can also inhibit the body's ability to absorb vitamin B1 and can cause magnesium loss. It can also interfere with iron absorption. (Remember that anemia can cause depression.) The link between vitamin B1, magnesium and mood is discussed in Chapter 17.

In conclusion, I believe a number of health problems can be relieved by simply cutting caffeine from the diet. I have talked to several people who have eliminated a number of mental and physical symptoms just by nixing caffeine and by adding a daily dose of B vitamins. For years, professionals in the health and nutrition field have warned against the side effects of caffeine. Only recently, has the scientific community taken notice. Below are two examples of recent concern over caffeine use.

NURSES, SUICIDE AND CAFFEINE

A recent study conducted at Warneford Hospital in Oxford, England, reported that nurses are at a higher than normal risk for suicide and that this increased risk has been statistically related to extent of caffeine consumption. While other factors certainly come into play, consuming caffeine played a major role in determining the risk of suicide among these nurses.

CAFFEINE AFFECTS MELATONIN

Researchers at the Department of Psychology at Bowling Green State University recently found that circadian rhythms were altered by caffeine, suggesting that the secretion of melatonin is changed when we consume caffeine. Melatonin manipulation could certainly contribute to the sleep/depression link, and if you suffer from SAD (seasonal affective disorder), using caffeine could make your symptoms worse.

Alcohol and Mood

Alcohol provides another major piece in the depression puzzle for many individuals. New study findings report that approxi-

The Devastating Alcohol Factor

Alcohol not only manipulates mood and sets up the brain for depressive illness, it also puts enormous stress on other body systems, impacting behavior. For example, using alcohol can create B vitamin, amino acid and mineral deficiencies. And you don't have to drink large quantities of alcohol to deplete stores of vitamin B. Consistently drinking even small quantities of alcohol can result in the malabsorption of vitamin B1, B2 and folic acid—all considered crucial nutrients to maintain mental health. In addition, other nutrients like vitamins B6 and C are destroyed by an alcohol by-product produced in the liver. This by-product is formed every time you drink. In fact, much of the nerve damage seen in alcoholics is the result of a thiamine deficiency (vitamin B1). Moreover, minerals such as zinc, calcium and magnesium are excreted more readily in the urine when alcohol is present in the bloodstream. Some recent studies have suggested that alcohol also decreases the metabolism of certain brain amines (like serotonin) formed from tyrosine.

mately 30 percent of people with major depression and 60 percent of people with bipolar depression abuse alcohol and drugs. These statistics reinforce the notion that addiction may reflect a genetic brain malfunction linked to depression. I've already discussed the fact that people with depression are twice as likely to be addicted to nicotine compared to those with no mood disorders. It seems that the same trend applies to alcohol use as well.

Alcohol may be the most devastating drug among our modern-day repertoire of addictive chemicals. Alcoholism is a major health problem and the third leading cause of death in this country. There are twelve million alcoholics in America today—not to mention the additional millions who are considered heavy drinkers. Alcohol has exacted an enormous financial, physical and emotional toll on our society.

Why is alcohol so dangerous? Alcohol detrimentally affects the brain, mood and our ability to function (see sidebar). It's that simple. And one reason that more women than men are alcoholics may be due to the large number of women who struggle with depression; consequently, they are more prone to reach for a drink.

Like any mind-altering drug, it is easy to become dependent on alcohol to achieve a sense of well-being or relaxation. If you drink to feel better, then you're a prime candidate for addiction. What is particularly troubling is that alcohol prevents you from confronting your depression. It only serves to potentiate the paralyzing effects of depressive illness.

Note: A recent study has found that using alcohol can impair the action of antidepressant drugs. Even mild use of alcohol can impair your response to all antidepressant medications.

Environmental Hazards to the Brain

There are a number of other brain hazards that are not ingested. Andrew Weil, M.D., who I believe has the ideal approach to using the best of both the conventional and natural treatment world has said, "Be wary of all the chemicals in your life." We live in a world teeming with hidden poisons, toxins and carcinogens. Be assured that these chemicals find their way into brain tissue and can alter both behavior and personality.

For example, chronic exposure to certain compounds and heavy metals can produce bizarre changes in mental outlook and behavior. A number of everyday solvents are also capable of interfering with brain cell biochemistry. In addition, certain paints, varnishes and virtually any toxic chemical or fume is capable of producing a mood disorder.

People who routinely work with paints and varnishes, refinery workers, people who manufacture or use pesticides, and people who routinely handle fuel may be at risk for developing personality changes, panic disorders, irritability and depression.

In addition, engaging in potentially lethal habits like sniffing glue, gasoline, cleaning fluid and nitrous oxide can also create mental disorders. The initial euphoria that results from these

244 • SOLVING THE DEPRESSION PUZZLE

kinds of activities turns into conduct-disordered behavior.
Exposure to these kind of chemicals creates abnormal behavior
that can be misinterpreted as a psychiatric disorder, not to mention the life-threatening nature of these habits. The bottom line is
not to underestimate the negative effects of exposing yourself to
toxic substances.

CARBON MONOXIDE

Carbon monoxide can damage the hippocampus area of the
brain, which can cause depression and changes in behavior.
Carbon monoxide, which comes from car exhaust, tobacco smoke
and wood burning, is a colorless and odorless gas. If you work in a
parking garage or have a faulty automobile exhaust system, you
may be getting slow doses of this poison. Carbon monoxide robs
oxygen from the body—including the brain. Brain cells are the
most sensitive to any kind of oxygen deprivation. As a result, if
your brain is oxygen starved, psychiatric symptoms can occur. Like
so many other conditions that can cause behavioral symptoms,
carbon monoxide poisoning can be easily misdiagnosed as schizophrenia or psychotic depression.

PESTICIDES

Organophosphate insecticides can have the same effect on the
nervous system as nerve gas used in chemical warfare. If you are
consistently exposed to these chemicals you can become irritable,
tense, anxious, restless, depressed and emotionally withdrawn.
This family of insecticides inhibits acetylcholinesterase, an essential enzyme in the brain.

METALS AND BRAIN CELLS

The connection between heavy metal exposure and depression
is also well documented. Of the naturally occurring elements,
sixty-nine are metals, and today, our metal usage has become more
clever and sophisticated. Metals are found in fuels, medicines,

makeup, hair spray, kitchen cleaners, herbicides and insecticides, and the recent link between aluminum salts and Alzheimer's still looms as a distinct possibility. (We routinely ingest aluminum in salt, some antacids, and cake mixes, just to name a few sources.)

Ingesting or breathing lead, mercury or radioactive metals can also wreak havoc with the human body and create psychiatric mayhem in the mind. The brain is hypersensitive to these metals, and strange behavior may be the first clue that poisoning has occurred. In addition, zinc, lead, mercury, bismuth, aluminum, bromides, lithium, thallium and organophosphates can all cause clinical depression. One report links high levels of a mineral called vanadium to depression, but taking vitamin C helps to detoxify vanadium. Refer to the detoxification plan at the end of this chapter for more detail on how to clear your system of metal and mineral toxicity.

Mineral Imbalance

Too little or too much of certain minerals can also create mental problems. For example, if you overuse diuretics, you can develop a sodium or potassium deficiency serious enough to cause harmful symptoms. A lack of iron can make you feel depressed and irritable, while too much iron can be life threatening. If you have a thyroid disorder or pancreatitis, you can develop serious symptoms of calcium overload in the blood, which can manifest itself as depression or psychiatric illness. A condition referred to as "manganese madness" can occur in people who work in manganese mines or steel foundries where manganese dust is inhaled. In these cases, depression is typical.

Protecting Yourself

One very good reason for taking vitamin and mineral supplements in dosages higher than the RDA recommends is to protect ourselves against hidden environmental poisons we encounter

246 • SOLVING THE DEPRESSION PUZZLE

each day. We've all heard the term free radicals, which refers to molecules that are extremely reactive because they contain an unpaired electron. Free radicals cause damage to the human body by destroying cellular structures. Common sources of free radicals are car exhaust, herbicides, pesticides, drugs, cigarette smoke, radiation, food additives, industrial waste and polluted air.

If you take an antioxidant supplement daily, you can help neutralize the devastating biological effects of free radicals. Antioxidant compounds include vitamin E, vitamin C, vitamin A, beta carotene, bioflavonoids and alpha lipoic acid.

The Last Word on Chemicals and Mood

If you are suffering from unexplained depression, examine your home and work environment, and make sure that you are not continually exposed to harmful toxins without protection. Take a good antioxidant supplement daily, and if you are trying to get rid of the toxic effects of nicotine, alcohol or caffeine, use the following detoxification plan in combination with the core protocol for depression.

Supplement Game Plan for Detoxification (Use with Core Protocol)

WATER
Typical dosage: Drink 8 to 10 glasses of water with fresh-squeezed lemon juice daily

VITAMIN A
Typical dosage: 10,000 IU daily

BETA CAROTENE
Typical dosage: 15,000 IU daily

GRAPESEED OR PINEBARK EXTRACT
Typical dosage: 200 to 300 mg daily

MILK THISTLE OR SILYMARIN
Typical dosage: 50 to 200 mg daily

QUERCETIN
Typical dosage: 500 mg three times daily

APPLE CIDER VINEGAR
Typical dosage: Take 1 to 2 tablespoons mixed in water daily

VITAMIN E
*Note: This can replace the dosage recommendation for vitamin E
found in the Core Protocol*
Typical dosage: 400 to 800 IU daily

VITAMIN C
*Note: This can replace the dosage recommendation for vitamin C
found in the Core Protocol*
Typical dosage: Take 1 to 4 grams daily

CHAPTER 17

Vitamins and Minerals: Key Mood Boosters

A STUDY PUBLISHED in a 1999 edition of *Psychosomatic Medicine* states:

> Although evidence for the use of vitamins and amino acids as sole agents for psychiatric symptoms is not strong, there is intriguing preliminary evidence for the use of folate, tryptophan, and phenylalanine as adjuncts to enhance the effectiveness of conventional antidepressants. More research should be conducted on these and other natural products for the prevention and treatment of various psychiatric disorders.

I was rather amused when I read this quote. I can tell you that I personally feel that there is ample evidence that the compounds mentioned in this quote, as well as others, can help you beat your depression. Throughout the first part of this book, I have reiterated the importance of nutrition in treating depression. Vitamin and mineral supplementation, in particular, have been discussed as essential to treating depression naturally. In this section, I want to discuss the benefits of each mood-boosting mineral and vitamin in more detail. Vitamin and mineral levels in the body could be a piece in your depression puzzle, and supplementation may be a possible solution—without the side effects of drugs.

Key Vitamins for Mood Elevation

In the 1960s, a psychiatrist found that adding megavitamin therapy to the standard medical treatment of three schizophrenic patients had striking results. Each was placed on a low blood sugar diet supplemented with megadoses of niacin in combination with Vitamin C, B6 and E. One patient in particular improved so dramatically that her life took a dramatic upturn and electric shock treatments were no longer necessary. This psychiatrist eventually developed a private practice that uses nutritional therapy consisting of diet and vitamins to treat patients who would otherwise be taking mood-altering drugs.

In fact, few people are aware of studies like one published in a 1999 edition of the *Journal of Epidemiology* reporting that alpha-tocopherol, or vitamin E, actually stopped the progression of depression in elderly men when combined with certain cholesterol levels.

Unfortunately, doctors who are willing to use vitamin therapy are few. Chances are, if you ask your physician to use vitamin therapy for your depression, he'll brush off the idea. Although this book does not propose that all mental disorders are the result of nutritional deficiencies, in many cases, vitamins play a profound role in facilitating a cure. We do know that some psychologically disturbed individuals suffer from the abnormal metabolism of one or more vitamins, minerals, amino acids or fatty acids. Such abnormal metabolisms can lead to nutrient deficiencies. Let's look at some brief profiles of certain vitamins and minerals that are considered especially brain friendly.

The B-Complex Vitamins

B vitamins are particularly important for brain health. Not only do they provide vital nutrients for brain function, a lack of any one of them can produce depression, anxiety, irritability, lethargy and fatigue. People with bipolar and clinical depression have responded to B vitamin therapy, suggesting that their illness may have been due to a lack of these vitamins. Interestingly, a vitamin B deficiency can also be a side effect of depression, especially since many depressed individuals eat poorly. In fact, it's sometimes difficult to tell which came first—the depression or the deficiency.

Keep in mind also that B vitamins are easily destroyed by other compounds. Penicillin, cigarette smoke, and a whole host of pollutants and toxic chemicals can wipe out vitamin B stores in the body. The widespread contamination of our environments by vitamin B antagonists may be responsible, in part, for the ever escalating incidence of depression. Other substances or factors that destroy B vitamins include:

- alcohol
- antacids
- anticonvulsants
- barbiturates
- caffeine
- cooking heat
- diuretics
- fever
- heat
- high-protein diets
- oxalic acid
- rancid fats and oils
- some laxatives
- stress
- tobacco
- aluminum
- antibiotics
- aspirin
- birth control pills
- chlorine
- cortisone
- estrogen
- food processing
- heavy metals
- mineral oil
- radiation
- some antidepressant drugs
- some sleeping pills
- sugar
- ultraviolet light

If you decide to take vitamin B supplements for depression, be advised that when you first start, you may experience an initial period where you feel even worse. For reasons that remain unclear, an initial rise in B6 levels (for example) can cause your depression to intensify. In these cases, experimenting with reduced dosages may be necessary.

There are several theories suggesting that brain amines may become more unbalanced as the body adjusts to a rise in certain vitamins, and that enzyme malfunctions may react negatively to the presence of the vitamin. These reasons are purely speculative; however, anyone who decides to take any supplements should do so with their health care provider's approval.

Remember also that creating a working equilibrium between all vitamins and minerals is the ultimate goal. In general, B vitamins tend to work best together as a group; however, when it comes to targeting depression, you may need stronger doses of specific B vitamins than what is offered in a B-complex supplement. Let's go over the best of the B vitamins for improving mood and decreasing the risk of depression.

VITAMIN B1

Also known as thiamine, a lack of this vitamin can cause many types of psychological disorders. It's important to understand that thiamin deficiencies can easily occur as a result of our excessive

B Vitamins and Geriatric Blues

Researchers at the Department of Psychiatry of Harvard Medical School conducted a study which found that adding vitamins B1, B2 and B6 to the diets of older individuals on drugs for depression greatly enhanced their response to the drugs. What was really fascinating is that the B12 levels in these patients also increased without specific supplementation. They concluded that the B-complex vitamins should be considered for treatment of geriatric depression.

consumption of refined white flour and sugar foods. When we eat these foods, we usually aren't eating enough whole grains (that supply us with thiamin).

Dosage: Take 100 mg daily. The allithiamine form of vitamin B1 is fat-soluble.

VITAMIN B2

Vitamin B2, also known as riboflavin, helps keep our antioxidant enzymes in tip-top shape. While specific studies linking this vitamin to mental health are lacking, it makes up an integral part of B-complex supplements and should not be ignored. Antioxidant activity in brain cells is very important. In fact, new evidence suggests that some individuals become depressed because their brain cells are slow to rid themselves of toxins and old chemicals.

Dosage: Take 50 mg of vitamin B2 daily. Be aware that this is the vitamin that gives your urine the dark yellow color when excreted through the kidneys. There is no danger in this.

VITAMIN B3

While we routinely use niacin (vitamin B3) to help lower cholesterol levels, many people don't know that this vitamin is necessary for the proper metabolism of tryptophan to serotonin in the brain. Recently, niacin supplementation has been used to help people who are withdrawing from addictive substances like drugs or alcohol. Niacin actually dilates blood vessels and improves circulation, actions which may explain its positive effect on mood. While its clinical credentials for depression are not as impressive as the other B vitamins, its presence in your supplement program is vital. It helps to balance out the other B vitamins, so they will render an optimal effect.

Dosage: 400 mg taken twice daily. Excessive niacin can cause flushing of the skin, which looks much like a good case of hives.

This effect is due to its effect on blood vessels and will usually disappear within thirty minutes. You may want to try time-released niacin to avoid this effect; another form of niacin that does not cause skin flushing is called inositol hexaniacinate. You should not take niacin if you have a peptic ulcer or gout.

VITAMIN B6

Vitamin B6 (pyridoxine/pyridoxal-5-phosphate) is the stellar B vitamin when it comes to controlling mood and behavior. A lack of this vitamin can cause irritability, which is often seen in manic depressives. Moreover, B6 can be used to treat PMS, birth control pill-induced irritability, and postpartum depression. Many people who suffer from these disorders also have a B6 deficiency.

One study of fifteen depressed, pregnant women revealed that they all suffered from some degree of vitamin B6 deficiency. Interestingly, several other studies have found that some women who take birth control pills and become depressed after starting them also have low levels of B6.

Scientific evidence that B6 can effectively treat depression also came from an English study that carefully observed twenty-two depressed women who were all taking birth control pills. Because birth control pills can deplete the body of vitamin B6, researchers assumed that the deficiency was related to the onset of depression. Half of these women were found to be deficient in vitamin B6, and when given supplements, they experienced relief from their depression.

Researchers at the University of Miami School of Medicine discovered that vitamin B6 supplementation may even make periods of grief or bereavement easier. They found that if you are B6 deficient, your reaction to sorrow may be more intense and debilitating. They concluded that higher vitamin B6 levels can help to prevent psychological distress in times of bereavement. Why? Because vitamin B6 is a cofactor for 5-hydroxytryptophan decarboxylase—the enzyme necessary to make serotonin.

In light of these studies, the *British Journal of Psychiatry* concluded that "more attention should be paid to assessing the pyridoxine (vitamin B6) status of the mentally ill in the hope of detecting and correcting deficiencies." Research supports the fact that as many as 20 percent of people hospitalized for depression lack vitamin B6. What is troubling is that these people showed no physical signs of this deficiency.

Several other studies done at the Virginia Polytechnic Institute and State University and at the National Institute of Mental Health have confirmed that plasma levels of vitamin B6 were approximately 48 percent lower in depressed patients. While some doctors refute the validity of the vitamin B6 connection to severe depression, the statistics cannot be ignored or misinterpreted.

While vitamin B6 is readily available in most foods, deficiencies can result from taking certain drugs, including birth control pills. In addition exposure to a variety of pollutants and ingesting too much sugar or caffeine can inhibit its action. Several other studies done at the Virginia Polytechnic Institute and State University and at the National Institute of Mental Health have confirmed that plasma levels of vitamin B6 were approximately 48 percent lower in depressed patients.

Women who suffer from postpartum depression have a higher risk for developing a vitamin B deficiency. Some women become deficient in Vitamin B6 during the course of their pregnancy. Consequently, after the baby is born they experience an intense period of melancholia. In some cases, where a lack of vitamin B6 was not a factor, deficiencies in vitamin B12 or folate were discovered. At any rate, keeping the body supplied with adequate amounts of the B vitamins is essential to preventing or treating certain cases of unexplained depression.

It is also vital that we all remember that blood and urine tests don't always conclusively represent what may be going on in brain biochemistry. It has been pointed out that a vitamin B6 deficiency could conceivably exist in the brain, even when blood or urine levels look normal. People who have abnormal enzyme function in the brain may require unusually high amounts of vitamin B6 to function normally. This would explain why some people develop depression, even if they consume adequate supplies of vitamin B6.

While vitamin B6 is readily available in most foods, deficiencies can result from taking certain drugs—including oral contraceptives, exposure to a variety of pollutants, and ingesting too much sugar or caffeine. Ironically, MAO inhibitors, which are antidepressant medications, also deplete vitamin B6 reserves.

Dosage: Vitamin B6 supplementation can be a bit tricky, and high dosages taken over long periods of time may result in numbness of the fingers and/or toes. So, do not take any more than recommended. If you are taking extra B6, take it with the other B-complex vitamins to achieve a balance. Also, try to use the pyridoxal-5-phosphate form. It seems to be more bioavailable and look for an active coenzyme form. If you experience tingling or numbness in the toes or fingers, reduce the dosage immediately. The dosage range for vitamin B6 is from 10 mg per day to 250 mg. (Note that 50 mg is usually enough for most people; however, with depression, you should probably start with 100 mg daily.)

VITAMIN B12

A deficiency of vitamin B12 has been directly linked to a number of different mental illnesses including serious psychotic behavior. In fact, the first symptom of low B12 levels can be a disruption in thinking or behavior. In several studies that dealt with people suffering from manic depression, supplementation with intravenous B12 injections normalized behavior. Some doctors even believe that a vitamin B12 deficiency may be the true cause of manic or depressive symptoms in many cases. There is no doubt that B12 is vital for proper brain and nerve function.

Keep in mind that this member of the B-complex family is difficult to absorb in digestion, especially in older people, so deficiencies can easily occur. In addition, since this vitamin is supplied in meats, vegetarians often suffer deficiencies as well. An article in the *American Journal of Psychiatry* recommended that a B12 deficiency should be suspected in all patients with severe psychiatric symptoms. For our purposes, there is no question that vitamin B12 supplementation should be used to combat depression.

Dosage: Take 250 to 500 mcg (mcg) per day of vitamin B12 in sublingual tablets. In general, the sublingual or nasal forms of this vitamin are preferred. In extreme circumstances, doctors can also give shots of several thousand mcg. (No adverse side effects to very large amounts seem to have been reported.) In her book *The Way Up From Down*, Dr. Patricia Slagle recommends putting a B12 tablet under your tongue first thing in the morning to ward off depressive feelings.

It's easy enough to supplement one's diet with B vitamins, which have no harmful side effects and are relatively inexpensive. Women who take the pill should be advised by their physicians that taking B vitamins can help eliminate depressive side effects that sometimes occur. Get yourself a good supply of B vitamins, and take them for the rest of your life.

FOLIC ACID (FOLATE)

Folic acid, or folate, is another essential nutrient for treating depression. It works synergistically with vitamin B12 and contributes to neurotransmitter production in the brain. A deficiency of folic acid can also cause you to feel depressed. Folic acid is a member of the vitamin B family and is absolutely essential for the proper functioning of the brain and central nervous system. Research done at the Royal Victoria Hospital in Montreal clearly supports the fact that if you become deficient in folic acid and get depressed, taking supplements can make you feel entirely better.

Green leafy vegetables are the main source of folic acid; however, high cooking temperatures destroy over half the available vitamin content. Due to its vulnerability to heat, folic acid deficiencies are common. Some physicians actually assess your overall nutritional status by checking your levels of folic acid. That's how vital it is.

And if you think you're getting enough folic acid from your diet, think again. Poor eating, which includes many weight-reducing diets, can be responsible for low levels. In addition, taking aspirin, barbiturates, anticonvulsants, oral contraceptives and other drugs can inhibit the absorption of folic acid in the body. The early signs of a folic acid deficiency are fatigue and lethargy. Later on, depression, burning feet, and restless leg syndrome can occur.

Blood levels of folic acid are frequently low in a significant number of depressed individuals. As many as 30 percent of psychiatric patients are low in folic acid. In one study, 67 percent of elderly patients admitted to a psychiatric facility were deficient in folic acid. Unfortunately, it is rarely addressed.

Furthermore, folic acid levels not only affect mood, but also boost the action of antidepressants. A recent study by two Harvard Medical School doctors found that patients with the lowest folate levels have more depressive symptoms and don't respond as well to treatment. In a test of 213 adults with major depression, researchers discovered that those with low levels were less likely to benefit from eight weeks of treatment with fluoxetine (Prozac) than those with normal levels. You may remember that folic acid is a vitamin that is also now known for its importance in preventing spinal malformations in developing fetuses.

Dosage: Despite the tremendous good folic acid can do, manic depressives need to be careful about taking high doses of folic acid (probably in excess of 3,000 mcg per day), since it may intensify manic behavior. Large doses of folic acid also reduce the efficiency of anticonvulsants such as Depakote for epileptics and manic depressives.

Vitamin C and Bioflavonoids

Vitamin C and bioflavonoids also have mood-boosting properties and are needed to produce norepinephrine and serotonin in the brain. Bioflavonoids, in combination with vitamin C, provide the body with a very impressive defense system against oxidation or the breakdown of norepinephrine in brain cells. New studies also suggest that bioflavonoids promote better memory and reduce insomnia. And because bioflavonoids are nutrients that cannot be produced by the human body, they have to be obtained from foods or supplements. While RDA requirements for bioflavonoids are usually met by a decent diet, the therapeutic use of bioflavonoids holds tremendous promise for a variety of ailments including neurological disorders.

Bioflavonoids have the ability to pass through the blood-brain barrier, thereby serving as antioxidants to brain cells. Several scientific studies strongly suggest that antioxidants can help restore normal neurochemical balance in the brain following surgery or trauma. Oxidative stress is repeatedly cited and implicated in a wide variety of nervous system disorders. In fact, some experts now believe that brain cell toxicity may be the real cause of depression in many people.

Bioflavonoids are the chemical constituents of the pulp and rind of citrus fruits, green peppers, apricots, cherries, grapes, papayas, tomatoes and broccoli. Bioflavonoids are not really considered vitamins; however, their value is enormous. For one thing, they increase the body's ability to absorb vitamin C. It's important to always take vitamin C together with bioflavonoids since they greatly enhance each other.

Dosage: Look for ascorbic acid in tablet, capsule or powdered form. Buffered vitamin C is available and is easier on the stomach and less sour to the taste. Be aware of the fact that there are several expensive varieties of vitamin C, such as time released C or esterized varieties; however, there is not evidence that these more effective than plain old ascorbic acid, which is relatively inexpensive. It is essential to get a vitamin C supplement that contains bioflavonoids.

Minerals for Mood Elevation

Minerals are also intrinsically involved in the preservation of wellness and good mental health. In fact, without the proper array of minerals, all the vitamins in the world will do no good, and as I mentioned in the chapter on malnutrition and depression, mineral deficiencies can be much more common than you might think. Mineral-poor soil, diets low in fresh produce, and our exposure to stress and toxic chemicals can make any of us mineral-deficient.

Chromium

Chromium is a trace mineral that maintains normal blood sugar and helps to support the function of insulin. It is a part of the glucose tolerance factor (GTF) that helps to regulate the metabolism of sugar. There is some new evidence that this particular mineral may also work to maintain normal brain activities. For example, one study published in a 1999 issue of the *Journal of Clinical Psychiatry* reported that chromium supplementation actually made the effect of antidepressant drugs more powerful. Researchers at the Department of Psychiatry at the University of North Carolina School of Medicine found that chromium supplementation led to remission of depressive symptoms. Preliminary observations suggested that, in conclusion, chromium may potentiate the use of antidepressant drugs for certain kinds of depression.

While this study only dealt with people on drugs for depression, it also implies that chromium must play a previously unexplored role in brain chemistry. I also believe that because blood sugar and insulin play such a profound role in how we feel about life, taking chromium supplements is a good idea.

Dosage: Take 400 mcg of GTF chromium daily.

Calcium and Magnesium

Many experts also believe that calcium and magnesium have the power to help chase the blues away in some individuals. Ninety-nine percent of calcium is found in our bones and teeth, but the remainder of our calcium stores affect the nerves. In fact, a lack of calcium has been linked to irritability and depression.

While most of us may think we're getting enough calcium from dairy products, the truth is that up to 30 percent of the American population may be low in this crucial mineral, and even a relatively mild calcium deficiency can prompt all kinds of drastic behavioral changes.

In fact, the body is extremely sensitive to fluctuations in calcium levels. Brain cells cannot function normally if there is too little or too much calcium. Dr. August F. Daro, an obstetrician and gynecologist in Chicago, gives his depressed patients calcium and magnesium as a standard treatment. He states,

> [M]any depressed men and women are short on calcium and magnesium . . . I put them on a combination of 400 milligrams of calcium and 200 milligrams of magnesium a day. These minerals sedate the nervous system, and most of the depressed patients feel much better while taking them. Calcium and magnesium especially take care of premenstrual depression.

Most Americans don't get their RDA of magnesium either. A troubling situation considering that a magnesium deficiency can cause anxiety, insomnia (particularly premature waking), chronic fatigue, fibromyalgia, high blood pressure, PMS and depression. Magnesium supplementation is a good idea, especially for those suffering from a mood problem.

In fact, one study of forty-one unmedicated, psychiatric patients indicated that eleven women who had attempted suicide had significantly lower cerebrospinal fluid levels of magnesium than the other women. As a result, one cannot help but think that magnesium may be required to maintain normal serotonin activity in the brain. Comparable studies of other psychiatric patients who experienced depression, schizophrenia and sleep disturbances also pointed to low magnesium blood levels.

Interestingly, like phenylalanine, a lack of magnesium can create a chocolate craving. Taking magnesium supplements for PMS symptoms has been recommended to help stem the mood swings that typically occur in some women. In fact, changes in estrogen levels may affect magnesium levels, which may in turn, affect mood. It's also interesting to learn that depressed people who took lithium and improved also showed a rise in their magnesium levels, while the magnesium levels of those who tried lithium and stayed depressed remained the same.

Dosage: Magnesium is usually supplemented with calcium because the two minerals are absorbed better when taken together. The usual recommendation is two parts calcium to one part magnesium, which translates to 1,000 mg of calcium and 500 mg of magnesium. Keep in mind that higher doses of magnesium may be necessary for controlling PMS, fibromyalgia or depression. If you have trouble sleeping, take this supplement prior to bedtime. Also, although calcium carbonate is a common form of calcium, it is the least absorbable. I recommend using amino acid chelates, calcium citrate or hydroxapatite forms of calcium.

Mineral Balance

There is also considerable speculation that too much of one mineral and not enough of another can create depressed mental states. Some medical doctors believe that the most common mineral imbalance among people who are depressed is an excess of copper and a lack of zinc and manganese. In these cases, zinc and manganese are administered in combination with vitamin B6 to initiate the excretion of copper in the urine. If you suspect that this may be a problem, use chelated zinc.

CHAPTER 18

SAMe and Omega-3 Fats: New Fighters on the Depression Front

I've found that the chief difficulty for most people was to realize that they had really heard new things: that is things that they had never heard before. They kept translating what they heard into their habitual language. They had ceased to hope and believe there might be anything new.

PETER DEMIANOVICH OUSPENSKY

THIS CHAPTER WILL give you an overview of the latest natural sensation for depression called SAMe along with commentary on certain fatty acids and their very important connection to brain health. These supplements have been recommended throughout the book for their effects on mood. I decided to devote a whole chapter to describing how they work because I believe that this information will be helpful to you as you piece together your depression puzzle. Let's begin by looking at SAMe.

SAMe: An Introduction

SAMe (S-adenosylmethionine) recently hit American markets and can now be found in health food, drug and even grocery stores. In Europe, SAMe is available only by prescription and has been used to treat depression for years. Is it a legitimate treatment for depression? In my own research, I found over thirty-five scientific studies on SAMe. Several of these studies concluded that it works as well as antidepressant drugs with little or no side effects—a fact very few Americans are aware of.

Even more impressive is SAMe's ability to act more rapidly than drugs to elevate mood in many cases. Human trials found that people using SAMe actually felt better within a week rather than the four to six week required by most antidepressant drugs. However, like any new compound, while the initial test data is encouraging, more extensive studies are certainly needed. And like any prescription medication for depression, SAMe doesn't work for everyone. It's important to realize that this compound targets a different aspect of the brain. It's ability to detoxify brain cells make it act more as an antioxidant than a serotonin manipulator, although it is required to make brain chemicals like serotonin.

A Brain Antioxidant Defined

SAMe was discovered in 1952 in Italy. It is recognized as a biological compound found in every living cell, and it takes part in several reactions in the human body. Adults produce six to eight grams of SAMe daily. Most of it is made in the liver where it is utilized to detoxify the body of poisons that come in the form of drugs, alcohol, heavy metals, pesticides and solvents.

SAMe is vital to the manufacture and maintenance of neurotransmitter compounds like serotonin, norepinephrine, dopamine and phosphatidyl serine. It also has the ability to help these brain chemicals bind to their receptor sites, which enhances their tissue levels. Moreover, research tells us that increased levels of SAMe can boost detoxification in the body, which includes getting rid of not only poisons from our environment, but also old biochemical compounds made by the body itself. Old neurotransmitters are among these chemicals. The more efficiently we can sweep these from brain cells, the better new chemicals can function, helping to boost brain function and mood.

SAMe and Depression: The Impressive Data

We've established that the brain requires certain chemicals to function normally. When the level of these chemicals is disrupted, depression can occur. Moreover, subtle malfunctions in the way brain cells detoxify themselves may also be a factor. SAMe affects both. It works to detoxify brain cells and also plays a role in how certain neurotransmitters linked to mood are made and received.

It may provide a viable alternative to people with depression who cannot take prescription medications or don't want to deal with their side effects. For instance, according to statistics from the Substance Abuse and Mental Health Services Administration (SAMSHA), 53 percent of drug-related admissions to emergency rooms are due to overdoses of antidepressants, especially the tricyclic variety. SAMe does not have the same risks as prescriptions, which makes it infinitely more appealing.

And while the exact mechanism involved in mood elevation is not entirely understood, it is believed that SAMe has a positive effect on the membranes of brain cells, which sets into motion a series of cellular events impacting brain methyl groups. As a result, mood is elevated. Study after study confirms that SAMe is not only effective, it also comes with few side effects and is remarkably well tolerated, even in the elderly and psychologically disturbed patients.

SAMe Lauded by Scientists

Scientists at the Texas Tech University School of Medicine Department of Psychiatry came to similar conclusions:

> The antidepressant property of SAMe has been supported by several uncontrolled and controlled studies. Compared to standard

antidepressant agents, SAMe has fewer side effects and a shorter lag period. Future studies to delineate SAMe-responsive depression are warranted.

And at the University of California Irvine Medical Center, another study published in the *American Journal of Psychiatry* compared SAMe supplementation to imipramine (a prescription antidepressant drug) in a double-blind study involving nineteen patients who met textbook requirements for major depressive illness.

Italian studies also stressed that elderly people suffering from depression can greatly benefit from SAMe therapy. Moreover, Italian researchers reported that improvement occurred rapidly (in as little as five days) and lasted for months. They concluded that since SAMe readily gives off methyl groups and since it passes the blood brain barrier, it probably positively influences the biochemistry of the brain. Consequently, it may be regarded as a highly useful drug in the treatment of depressive illness.

How Does SAMe Compare with Prescription Antidepressant Drugs?

In 1994, research from Denmark concluded that SAMe supplementation showed a greater response rate when compared with a placebo, and it had an antidepressant effect comparable with that of standard tricyclic antidepressants. Recommendations of this study stated,

> The efficacy of SAMe in treating depressive syndromes and disorders is superior with that of placebo and comparable to that of standard tricyclic antidepressants. Since SAMe is a naturally occurring compound with relatively few side effects, it is a potentially important treatment for depression.

Drugs often come with undesirable side effects or toxicities even if they are effective. Moreover, some people who are depressed have other illnesses that preclude them from taking standard anti-depressant medicines. The remarkable nontoxic nature of SAMe coupled with its extraordinary effectiveness make it a very desirable therapeutic agent for these individuals. Scores of studies, of which only a few have been cited in this publication, support its dramatic antidepressant action.

SAMe Supplementation Can Potentiate Other Drug Therapies

Several studies have also shown that taking SAMe with antidepressant drugs like imipramine can actually boost their effect. In a double-blind clinical trial carried out to see if SAMe sped up the action of imipramine (IMI), sixty-three outpatients with moderate to severe depression were studied. The patients were evaluated every other day, and after two weeks, it was reported that depressive symptoms decreased earlier in the patients who were receiving SAMe with their imipramine than in those who were receiving the prescription drug alone.

SAMe for Depression in Alcoholics

A 1994 study found that SAMe not only treats depression commonly seen in alcoholics, but has a detoxifying effect as well. In a four-week trial, forty alcoholic patients with major depression received 600 mg of SAMe daily. After a week, patients were evaluated using the Hamilton Rating Scale for Depression, among other tests. Significant improvements were seen in most scores beginning on day fourteen and continuing through to the end of the study. Toxin levels also dramatically dropped and certain biochemical readings returned to normal. No adverse reactions were reported. Meanwhile, standard antidepressant therapy has often been unsuccessful in treating depression in alcoholics.

SAMe for Postpartum Depression

In 1993, a study was published showing that SAMe treatment markedly improved the moods of women who were experiencing anxiety, depression and hostility after the births of their babies after only ten days of treatment. The study continued for a total of thirty days, and its findings indicate that SAMe supplementation works for women who have trouble with postpartum depression or anxiety. It achieved its goal of relieving psychological distress in a relatively short period of time. And for women who may be nursing and can't take any medication, SAMe supplementation may offer a viable way to combat postpartum depression. This possibility should be reviewed by a physician before starting therapy.

Menopausal Distress and SAMe

Along similar lines, a strictly controlled trial studied eighty Swiss women between the ages of forty-five and fifty-nine suffering from clinical depression related to menopause or post-hysterectomy. They were given SAMe for one month. Not surprisingly, significant improvement in this group of women was recorded and side effects were listed as extremely mild and transient. Using SAMe for hormonally induced anxiety and depression opens up a whole host of possibilities for women who also suffer from severe PMS. The hormonal component to depression is only now emerging as part of a delicate biochemical balance that when disrupted, even in the slightest way, can cause depression, nervousness, irritability and insomnia.

Reasons to Use SAMe for Depressive Illness

Unquestionably, SAMe has been proven itself to be an effective treatment for various kinds of depression—with the exception of bipolar depression (manic depressive). One of the most impressive properties of SAMe is that improvement can be seen in as little as five days. It should be considered as a treatment for the following reasons:

• It has few, if any, side effects.
• It is fast-acting; improvement occurs rapidly.
• It is nontoxic.
• It is very effective.
• It is well tolerated, even by the elderly and mentally disturbed.

Folic Acid, Vitamin B12, SAMe and Psychiatric Illness

Interestingly, in order to make SAMe naturally in the human body, adequate levels of folic acid (folate), choline and vitamin B12 must be present. It seems like no coincidence that low levels of these same nutrients have been linked to various psychiatric disorders. What this suggests is that methylation of brain cells as it relates to nutrient intake may be playing more of a role in psychiatric illness than previously thought. A 1994 study conducted in New Zealand focused on the biochemistry of methylation in people who were mentally disturbed and concluded that boosting it may improve cognitive function in patients with dementia. What they found was that using SAMe helped to actually improve the myelination of nerves in the brain and to address faulty folate metabolism. What they also concluded from the their data was that impaired methylation in the brain can result from a variety of factors that impact a number of neurological and psychiatric disorders.

Fibromyalgia and SAMe

Furthermore, the mysterious link between fibromyalgia and depression is supported by new data on SAMe supplementation. Thousands of women who suffer from fibromyalgia may benefit from SAMe supplementation. Test results are very encouraging. One study in particular compared the effects of SAMe therapy for fibromyalgia against using TENS (transcutaneous electrical nerve simulation) and found that after six weeks of therapy, SAME supplementation outperformed TENS in a number of ways.

Data published in *American Journal of Medicine* concluded that SAMe treatment was justified in people with fibromyalgia because it improved depressive state and reduced the number of trigger points, thereby making it an effective and safe therapy in the management of primary fibromyalgia. What is particularly significant about these findings is that many women with fibromyalgia take tricyclic antidepressants. As mentioned earlier, SAMe works as well or better than these drugs and also offers people with fibromyalgia added benefits.

The Depression Component in Rheumatoid Arthritis

On a related note, another autoimmune disorder, rheumatoid arthritis, and the depression that often accompanies it may also be affected by SAMe supplementation. Rheumatoid is the most severe type of arthritis. The immune system of rheumatoid sufferers acts against the joints and surrounding tissue the same way it would attack an unwanted invader. Joints in the hands, feet and arms become extremely painful, stiff and eventually deformed. This type of arthritis can affect the entire body. Gout is another disorder associated with a type of arthritis in which uric acid, a waste product, accumulates as crystals in the joints and causes inflammation. While no data is available yet on the effect of SAMe in the disease process, we do know that it can help combat the depression which can accompany rheumatoid arthritis.

A double-blind study compared the efficacy and tolerability of SAMe with that of placebo in the treatment of depression in rheumatoid arthritic (RA) patients. Results showed a significant improvement in the depression in RA patients, and there was a significant difference between SAMe and placebo in all variables measured. In addition, no side effects were recorded with SAMe for treatment of depression.

How to Use SAMe

The customary dosage for SAMe is 600–1,200 mg per day. It is recommended that individuals start with 100 mg taken three times a day. If this does not seem adequate, take 200 mg three times daily on an empty stomach. It usually takes at least two weeks of therapy before results are obtained, but it can take as little as five days for changes to be observed.

Cautionary Measures When Considering SAMe

You should not start a new therapy or decrease or eliminate any medication you may be on without your doctor's approval. SAMe has caused some slight nausea in some people; therefore, taking it with fruit or other carbohydrates is recommended for anyone who suffers from this side effect. SAMe is considered to be a very safe substance. Anyone suffering from manic depression should not take SAMe.

Protection from Estrogen Buildup

When we talk about SAMe's ability to detoxify the body of poisons, we are also referring to the inactivation of estrogen through the process of methylation. We have only just begun to realize the profound impact that estrogen excess has on the female body. Everything from an increased risk for breast cancer to symptoms of PMS have been linked to levels of circulating estrogen. Moreover, excess estrogen can cause the bile in the gallbladder to stagnate, increasing the risk of gallstones, and SAMe has already proven its ability to prevent this condition in women who were pregnant or using oral contraceptives. The ability of the body to excrete or breakdown estrogen has profound implications for all women, especially when it comes to determining mood and behavior.

Drawbacks of SAMe

One great disadvantage of SAMe is that it is expensive. Costs range somewhere between $2.50 to $4.50 per 400 mg pill. For some people, the cost of this supplement may prevent them from using it. If you decide to use SAMe as one of the supplements recommended in the core protocol program, look for tablets with enteric coatings to improve absorption, and purchase the new butanedisulfonate form if you can.

Be aware that there is some controversy over whether SAMe supplements provide adequate amounts of the compound, or even if it is usable. Also, there is no evidence that more expensive products are better. Hopefully, the price of SAMe will come down as its market grows.

Fatty Acids and the Brain

Did you know that 60 percent of the brain is made of fatty acids? Did you also know that Americans typically eat fats that are bad for the body and leave out the ones that benefit health? In addition, new research suggests that faulty fat metabolism can be at the heart of some cases of depression.

What does fat have to do with mood? Eating the wrong kind of fats can disrupt blood chemistry and impair the way we break down fats into fatty acids. Without the right fatty acids, virtually every body system can be compromised. In addition, the right fatty acids actually ensure the workings of brain cells in a number of ways. Yes, serotonin definitely plays a role in mood; however, if brain cell membranes fail to function as they should, all the serotonin in the world won't work to properly elevate mood. But eating the right kinds of fats helps to keep cell membranes in optimal condition. Unfortunately, Americans have not chosen wisely when it comes to good dietary fats. Moreover, modern food processing techniques can deplete the omega-3 fatty acids found in foods by as much as 90 percent.

Ironically, during the last two decades and for the sake of our heart health, many of us abandoned butter and cream for margarines and semi-solid fats. We have also turned to vegetable oils because we thought they were better for us. To our dismay, margarine may have replaced the saturated fat and cholesterol found in butter with something that may be much more menacing—many margarines contain trans-fatty acids (TFAs). In fact, the TFA composition of commercially prepared hydrogenated fats varies from 8 to 70 percent and comprises approximately 60 percent of the fat found in processed foods.

Americans consume over 600 million pounds annually of TFAs in the form of processed frying fats. Experts now believe that TFAs can increase the risk of heart disease by 27 percent when consumed as at least 12 percent of the total fat intake. TFAs also reduce production of prostaglandins (hormones that act locally to control all cell-to-cell interactions) and interfere with fatty acid metabolism. It only stands to reason that if our brain cells rely on good lipids to function properly, many of us are in trouble.

Trans-fatty acids not only contribute to plaque accumulation in our arteries, but also disturb delicate brain chemistry, which can have a whole myriad of negative effects. Eating these fats can also lead to a depletion of the very fatty acids we need to maintain our health called essential fatty acids (EFAs). Some health experts believe that the widespread consumption of trans-fatty acids (which are created when a liquid oil is converted into a solid stick) has greatly contributed to mood disorders. Most of us have grown up on diets full of hydrogenated or man-made fats that are produced with extended shelf lives. Even vegetable oils like corn and safflower oil are not the best choice.

To make matters worse, we have failed to consume enough omega-3 fatty acids, which come from foods like coldwater fish and compounds like DHA. If lipid metabolism contributes to mood, then it should be one of the first things a person corrects if they suffer from depression. Using essential fatty acid supplements, (from fish or flaxseed), switching from corn oil to olive oil (monounsaturated), and using butter sparingly are all smart fat choices for optimal health, especially mental health.

Omega-3 Fatty Acids: Fabulous Fats

Omega-3 fats are the ones we most need—and the ones we neglect most. The digit "3" refers to differences in the oil's chemical structure and describes its chain of carbon atoms. A major source of omega-3 fatty acids is called alpha-linolenic acid (ALA) and is found in flaxseed and canola oils, pumpkin, walnuts and soybeans. Fish oils such as salmon, cod and mackerel, contain two other important omega-3 fatty acids known as DHA (docosahexaenoic acid) and EPA (eicosapentaenoic acid). We'll discuss the benefits of DHA for depression in more detail in a later section of this chapter.

It is common knowledge that omega-3 fats help reduce the risk of heart disease, but few of us realize they can impact the brain as well. Once taken into the body, omega-3 fats are converted to prostaglandins, which are hormone-like compounds that regulate many of our metabolic functions. Again, nutritionists have long been aware of the value of these fats for cardiovascular health, but their link to mental health has recently turned some scientific heads. We now know that omega-3 fatty acids help to keep the composition of nerve cells in the brain healthy. A lack of these fats coupled with excess amounts of saturated fats can actually change the flexibility of brain cells, making them less efficient.

Fish Oil and Psychiatric Disorders

Could eating salmon everyday be as effective as Prozac for depression? We don't know if depression causes lower omega-3 levels, but we do know that diets deficient in omega-3 fats can put you at a higher risk for the disease. Moreover, if you're already vulnerable to depression, eating a diet that's lacking in these fatty acids may put you over the edge. According to recent studies, the omega-3 fatty acids found in fish oil may actually reduce the symptoms of a variety of psychiatric illnesses, including schizophrenia, bipolar disorder, and depression. Some of this new data was reported at a workshop sponsored by the National Institutes of Health (NIH).

One study conducted by Dr. Andrew Stoll at Harvard Medical School gave fourteen bipolar patients daily supplements of fish oil and found that nine reacted favorably compared with only three of sixteen patients receiving a placebo substance. Another study used eicosapentaenoic (EPA), an omega-3 fish oil component, and reported a 25 percent improvement in schizophrenic symptoms.

Another study, conducted by scientists at Ohio State University Medical Center found that these fatty acids affect immune cell function, and by doing so, may help to negate the damaging effects of mental stress on the body itself. A study published in a 1998 issue of the *Journal of Affective Disorders* reported that the DHA and omega-3 fatty acid found in fish oil is crucial for the proper transmission between nerve cells in the brain and to prevent damage from free radicals. They discovered that people with low levels of DHA had much more severe depression. They concluded with a rather dramatic statement that using omega-3 supplements may alleviate the symptoms of depression.

All in all, these studies showed a relationship between the severity of the depression and the level of omega-3 deficiency. Now, a more recent study has compared levels of omega-3 fats in healthy people and people diagnosed with depression. On average, levels of omega-3 fatty acids were 40 percent lower in patients suffering from depression.

DHA: A Special Omega-3 Fatty Acid

As we mentioned, one type of omega-3 fat is called DHA and is found in fish oil. It makes up 30 percent of certain brain cell membranes in healthy people. DHA (which can easily be mistaken for DHEA) is another nutrient that is vital to maintaining healthy brain structure and function. Experts now believe that using DHA in supplement form may have some very impressive health benefits for anyone with chronic depression.

DHA (docosahexaenoic acid) is the main fatty acid found in the retina of the eye and in the gray matter of the brain as well as being an omega-3 long-chain fatty acid. We've already established the

Vitamin D and Omega-3s for Seasonal Affective Disorder

If you suffer from SAD and add vitamin D to your omega-3 supplement, you may get optimal results. In a small study reported in a recent issue of *Psychopharmacology*, college students who took 400 IU of vitamin D during the winter reported feeling more energy and more mental alertness than those who took a placebo. Adding vitamin D to a good omega-3 supplement is a good idea for anyone battling the winter blues.

fact that omega-3 fatty acids are essential to brain health. Before we are born, we are supplied DHA through the placenta, and after birth we get it from breast milk, fish (tuna, salmon and sardines), red meats, animal organs, and eggs. You can see that many of the food sources of DHA are now on everybody's nix list, so the chances of inadequate DHA consumption is a real concern. In addition, studies published in the *European Journal of Clinical Nutrition* suggest that the DHA content of breast milk of U.S. women is among the lowest in the world, indicating that DHA supplementation is a good idea.

Low levels of DHA in breast milk are of particular concern. DHA is vital for the proper growth and functional development of the brain in infants, and the DHA-rich diet can improve learning ability. In fact, DHA deficiencies have been linked to learning disorders. Why? The brain favors DHA. In other words, brain cells prefer to take up DHA over other fatty acids, and they turn it over very rapidly. New studies suggest that our infants are not receiving enough DHA. As a result, they may be prone to attention deficit hyperactivity disorder, unipolar depression, and hostility.

DHA is also essential for good cardiovascular health. Interestingly, it is DHA deficiency in some people with heart disease that also makes them susceptible to depression. DHA has been the subject of numerous studies, and I believe it should be considered as part of a natural treatment program for depression. DHA supports nerve cells and plays a key role in the transmission of electrical signals between brain cells. It actually helps these cells stay flexible. Low levels of DHA have been linked to mood changes, memory loss, depression and Alzheimer's disease. Some researchers with the National Institutes of Health stated in a 1995 issue of the *American Journal of Nutrition* that the documented steady increase in the incidence of depression seen over the last 100 years may be linked to declining DHA consumption levels.

Like the other omega-3 fatty acids we talked about, a lack of DHA can also put women at a higher risk for postpartum depression, not to mention diseases like multiple sclerosis. Some experts believe that using long-chain polyunsaturated fatty acids, particularly DHA, may reduce the development of depression. DHA deficiencies starting in childhood may contribute to conditions like depression later in life. New studies have strongly suggested that hyperactivity in children can be related to a lack of good fatty acids like DHA in childhood diets. DHA also works to keep mental functions sharp and can help give you the edge when it comes to retaining facts, working out problems and the capacity to draw from memory.

When considering how to get optimal levels of DHA and other omega-3s, a good suggestion is to try eating at least one three-ounce serving of salmon per week. This provides almost two grams of omega-3 fatty acids. If eating fish on a regular basis is not realistic, then use a good omega-3 supplement. Flaxseed oil and fish oil are recommended. If you use fish oil, make sure to take it with your vitamin E supplement to prevent any oxidation.

CHAPTER 19

Using 5-HTP and Other Amino Acids to Fight Depression

Nature never breaks her own laws.
LEONARDO DA VINCI

SO FAR, SEVERAL therapies have been mentioned as possible treatments for depression. The success of each of these therapies depends on the causes of your depression. Testing different therapies is an integral part of the puzzle-solving process for piecing together solutions to your depression. As you begin testing different treatment programs, consider trying amino acid supplementation.

Amino acid therapy promises to become one of the more effective natural treatments for depression. There is significant evidence that using certain amino acids in therapeutic doses can boost brain levels of specific neurotransmitters required to prevent the onset of depression. In fact, one of the objectives of taking certain free-form amino acids is to initiate the production and concentration of serotonin and norepinephrine, two of the main mood-altering brain chemicals.

Amino acids are the basic building blocks of the 40,000 different proteins found in the body. Approximately twenty amino acids cannot be made by the body and can only be obtained through the diet. If you think that your diet is good and probably supplies you with plenty of amino acids, you may be surprised to learn that some studies have shown that only 60 percent of people who appear to be in good health have normal levels of all amino acids in their blood. One explanation for this is the fact that while you may be eating protein, it may not all be "usable" protein. In other words, even if you eat protein in abundance, much of that protein may be inferior. If you eat lots of fish, you may be getting enough usable protein, but if your diet is high in dairy products, you may assume you're getting plenty of protein when in fact, the availability of that particular kind of protein may be compromised.

In addition, because amino acids compete with each other for assimilation, eating protein foods does not necessarily mean that you will produce enough of the brain chemicals you need to sustain mood. Taking certain amino acids in supplement form, however, can create "precursor loading" in the brain that diet alone may not provide.

In one of its latest assessments of various alternative therapies, the American Psychiatric Association stated that amino acid therapies may have a great deal to offer in the treatment of psychiatric disease. One of the most effective amino acid compounds to recently take center stage for depression is called 5-hydroxytryptophan, or 5-HTP.

Tryptophan

Tryptophan is an amino acid found naturally in several foods, including cow's milk, eggs, poultry, and some nuts and seeds. Tryptophan that is obtained through the diet is usually converted by the brain into 5-HTP, which is then turned into serotonin. In fact, in order to make serotonin, brain cells must first make 5-HTP. Theoretically, if you provide your body with 5-HTP in the form of a supplement, you are giving your brain the advantage of having extra raw material to manufacture even more serotonin.

Tryptophan is also useful for depression triggered by carbohydrate cravings. As discussed previously, low serotonin levels in the brain may cause these cravings, but if tryptophan is available, serotonin levels should rise, helping to inhibit carbohydrate cravings. In a study of tryptophan and depression, the amino acid was administered to eleven patients so severely depressed that they required hospitalization. After a month, seven of the eleven had significantly less guilt, anxiety, insomnia and weight loss. The overall level of depression in the eleven, as determined by standard psychiatric tests, dropped by 38 percent. Interestingly, those that had the highest blood tryptophan levels improved the most.

Furthermore, serotonin deficiencies can be caused by a diet lacking tryptophan. One theory proposes that the high prevalence of corn, which is tryptophan-deficient, in the American diet may account for decreases in serotonin. The American consumption of corn has skyrocketed over the last fifty years. It's not uncommon to consume corn flakes, corn oil, corn oil margarines, cornstarch and corn meal in the form of chips and other products all in the same day. Corn, in many scenarios, has replaced whole wheat, which is a good natural source of tryptophan.

While meat also provides tryptophan, it contains a wide range of other amino acids that compete with each other. Consequently, a diet that is high in meat does not ensure increased levels of tryptophan in the brain. There's a constant struggle between tryptophan and other amino acids (e.g., tyrosine, phenylalanine, leucine, methionine and histidine) in brain chemistry. Eating a high-protein diet will increase blood levels of competing amino acids, making it possible for tryptophan levels in the brain to actually decrease. Unfortunately, after a batch of tryptophan supplements became contaminated with a particular microorganism, all tryptophan was pulled from American markets.

In fact, L-tryptophan was quite popular for treating depression and insomnia during the 1980s. In 1990, several deaths were attributed to the substance, and although these were later attributed to a contamination of the product (nonpharmaceutical grade) made by one particular manufacturer, these supplements were pulled from the market. However, L-tryptophan is currently available only by prescription in the United States. This may change in the near future.

5-HTP (5-hydroxytryptophan): An Introduction

Despite setbacks, a new form of tryptophan—a highly purified compound extracted from the West African medicinal plant *Griffonia simplicifolia*—has recently become available. 5-HTP (5-hydroxytryptophan) has been successfully used in clinical trials with people suffering from depression who are resistant to traditional therapies. Because it has the ability to boost serotonin without the negative side effects of antidepressant drugs, it is one of nature's best choices as a natural remedy for depression, anxiety and sleep disorders.

5-HTP is thought to provide brain cells with the required raw materials needed to make serotonin. In addition, it does not interfere with the normal metabolic processes of the brain and is free of the potentially serious side effects of the SSRI antidepressants, which include dry mouth, reduced libido, heart palpitations, tremors and anxiety.

Prozac, Zoloft, imipramine and other antidepressant drugs work by influencing serotonin levels and are all members of the selective serotonin re-uptake inhibitors (or SSRIs) class of drugs. They work by increasing serotonin levels indirectly. In other words, by blocking a process that inactivates serotonin, these drugs artificially keep its levels up. In so doing, these drugs interfere with the brains natural chemical checks and balance system.

Often referred to as "Nature's Prozac," 5-HTP theoretically increases the production of serotonin on a cellular level. Like other natural antidepressants such as SAMe and St. John's wort, 5-HTP has been used primarily in Europe, where physicians prescribe it for depression and insomnia as well. I might add here that because 5-HTP seems to work for appetite control, insomnia, anxiety and depression, the undeniable link between these disorders is once again reinforced.

5-HTP for Anxiety Attacks

In a 1990 study conducted in Holland, twenty patients with

panic disorder took 5-HTP (60 mg intravenously). None of these patients showed an increase in depressive symptoms or anxiety following treatment. By contrast, nine patients in the control group reported a depressed mood. Interestingly, blood tests showed that circulating levels of melatonin increased after the 5-HTP treatments, a fact which may help explain why 5-HTP is also prescribed for insomnia.

5-HTP and Insomnia

A Norwegian study reported that 5-HTP positively impacts sleep patterns by increasing the levels of serotonin that prompt sleep. Serotonin is needed to produce melatonin—a hormone we've already talked about that regulates sleeping and waking cycles. Cats were injected with 5-HTP (40 mg/kg body weight) or L-tryptophan. Both substances were able to produce a deep sleeping state.

5-HTP for Depression

In a 1991 Swiss study, patients diagnosed with clinical depression were given either 150 mg of fluvoxamine (a standard antidepressant drug) or 100 mg of 5-HTP, three times daily. The test subjects were evaluated every two weeks using standard psychological tests for clinical depression. After six weeks, both groups showed some improvement. The 5-HTP group, however, had a larger percentage of improved patients and a slightly higher degree of improvement. The therapeutic effect of 5-HTP appeared to become greater as time passed.

5-HTP Compared to Antidepressant Drugs

Another report compared the results of three studies involving 5-HTP and imipramine (a standard antidepressant drug). All three trials showed no difference in the effect of the two substances. In other words, 5-HTP appeared to perform as well as the conventional drug—without the dry mouth and tremors typically seen in people using imipramine.

And in a six-week trial, sixty-three people were given either 5-HTP or full doses of a European antidepressant called Luvox (similar to Prozac). Researchers found that 5-HTP rendered the same antidepressant benefits as Luvox, with fewer and less severe side effects.

5-HTP for Weight Loss

A 1992 study of obese test subjects conducted in Italy found that 5-HTP produced significant weight loss. 5-HTP supplementation appeared to help patients reduce their carbohydrate intake by inhibiting their desire to eat carbohydrates. In addition, it produced a feeling of "early satiety." In other words, they stopped eating earlier because they felt full. Consequently, their food intake was reduced, and they lost weight. With no dietary changes, people in the group taking 5-HTP lost an average 3.1 to 3.7 pounds during the six-week study. The researchers concluded that their findings together with the good tolerance of 5-HTP suggest that 5-HTP may safely be used to treat obesity. Naturally, the link between serotonin levels and hunger is a profound one as illustrated by the dramatic success of drugs like Phen-Fen, which led to substantial weight loss but did so by putting health in jeopardy.

5-HTP and Migraine Relief

There is some evidence that 5-HTP may be helpful with migraines. A Spanish study compared the use of 5-HTP and methysergide, which is a standard migraine drug. A significant number of both test study groups showed improvement in migraines. Seventy-five percent of the methysergide group and 71 percent of the 5-HTP group found relief. The 5-HTP produced nearly the same benefits as a standard migraine drug. In addition, the study showed that 5-HTP was particularly good for reducing the intensity and duration of the migraines rather than their frequency. Naturally, 5-HTP produced fewer side effects than the drug, and if you have migraines, 5-HTP may be used as a preventive compound. Once again, the effect of this amino acid compound on brain-related conditions supports its action on neurochemistry.

How Much 5-HTP Should I Take?

The typical recommended dosage of 5-HTP for depression is 25 to 50 mg daily, although you can take up to 100 mg daily in two divided doses. Don't take 5-HTP with other antidepressants or monoamine oxidase (MAO) inhibitors. If you go over 100 mg daily, you could experience nausea or headaches. Vitamin B6 should also be taken on the same day as 5-HTP because its presence is necessary to convert 5-HTP into serotonin.

Generally speaking, 5-HTP appears to be safe when used as directed. Side effects appear to be limited to the usual occasional, mild digestive distress and allergic reactions. In addition, 5-HTP is made by a completely different manufacturing process (by using a plant rather than a bacteria), and the risk of contamination is substantially lower. Be aware, however, that in September of 1998, the FDA released a report stating that some commercial 5-HTP preparations may contain bacteria. The issue is still unresolved, and the safe use of 5-HTP for young children, pregnant or nursing mothers, and those with liver or kidney disease has not been established.

Make sure you consult a qualified health practitioner before taking 5-HTP or natural L-tryptophan, particularly if you are currently taking any prescription medications. People with heart conditions or asthma should be careful because elevated serotonin levels may affect these disorders. Don't take a tryptophan supplement without your doctor's consent if you have Parkinson's disease, cancer, autoimmune disease, lung or liver diseases, anorexia, allergies, diarrhea, sickle cell anemia or hemophilia.

Tyrosine

Tyrosine, like tryptophan, plays a significant role in boosting brain neurotransmitters directly responsible for mood. L-tyrosine is an amino acid that serves as a precursor to the neurotransmitters norepinephrine and dopamine, which have been shown to be deficient in many manic depressives during their depressed cycles. The supplementation of this amino acid may help the body to form more of these substances during times of emotional stress. L-tyrosine can help mood by boosting the body's production of adrenaline, which causes a rise in dopamine levels. If a lack of tyrosine exists, insufficient levels of norepinephrine can also result, causing dips in mood.

Several doctors and psychiatrists have referred to tyrosine as a valuable treatment for ordinary depression and for the mood swings associated with PMS. In his book, *A Different Kind of Healing*, Oscar Janiger, M.D., comments:

> I've had great results with tyrosine. It's like a natural antidepressant and is a precursor to the neurotransmitter norepinephrine. Once the right dosage is determined, it usually works really well for people with mild depression or severe mood swings, especially if you add B vitamins.

The *American Journal of Psychiatry* relates a case in which a thirty-year-old woman, who had suffered for several years from depression and had actually become worse with drug therapy, finally tried tyrosine. A team of doctors from Boston and Cambridge gave her tyrosine supplements. The article reports that after only two weeks, her condition improved dramatically. She felt better than she had in years and showed striking improvement in mood, self esteem, sleep, energy level, anxiety and somatic (physical) complaints.

Cases such as this one may be challenged by some doctors who would assume her improvement was a result of the placebo effect. This same woman, however, was given a placebo as a substitute for tyrosine without her knowledge. After one week, her depression began to return. After eighteen days, she was more severely depressed than she had been prior to taking the tyrosine.

Dosage: Take tyrosine on an empty stomach with some fruit juice. It can raise blood pressure in some people, so don't use it if you have hypertension. Start at 500 mg daily and work up to 1,000 mg over four weeks.

DL-Phenylalanine (DLPA)

Phenylalanine is another naturally occurring amino acid found in protein foods. Like tyrosine, supplementation with phenylalanine appears to significantly boost mood. It is commonly used by practitioners in combination with St. John's wort for maximum results.

Phenylalanine is considered a natural antidepressant like tyrosine and tryptophan. It acts as a precursor to the amines that make up neurotransmitters in the brain. According to Jose A. Yaryura-Tobias, M.D., phenylalanine converts to phenylethylamine in the body, which is a natural antidepressant compound. L-phenylalanine can actually convert to tyrosine, and it also contributes to the formation of 2-PEA, which is believed to be closely tied with norepinephrine.

Some studies show that depressed people lack 2-PEA, and it has also been shown to be deficient in some manic depressives. As we have discussed previously, 2-PEA or phenylethylamine is also present in chocolate and marijuana. (So you won't get confused about the "DLPA," designation, know that phenylalanine exists in two forms that are mirror images of each other. These two forms are known as D- and L-phenylalanine. The combined DL form or (DLPA) is the product most commonly available in stores.)

DLPA COMPARED TO AN ANTIDEPRESSANT DRUG

A 1978 study compared the effectiveness of D-phenylalanine with the antidepressant drug called imipramine, given in doses of

100 mg daily. The study involved sixty patients who were randomly assigned to either one group or the other and followed carefully for thirty days. The results in both groups were statistically equal; however, DLPA appeared to work more rapidly than the prescription drug, producing significant improvement in two weeks. Another double-blind study assessed twenty-seven test subjects, half of whom received DLPA and the other half imipramine in full doses of 150 to 200 mg. Data revealed that after thirty days of treatment, the two groups had improved by the statistical margin.

Dosage: Most health care providers prescribe 400 to 800 mg daily of DL-phenylalanine, divided into two or three daily doses. Start with a low dose and work up. Take it on an empty stomach with a little fruit juice. Phenylalanine is thought to be safe, although comprehensive, long-term safety studies have not been conducted. Side effects are rare, although increased anxiety, headache and even mild hypertension have been reported when higher doses of phenylalanine are used.

Also, don't use phenylalanine if you have the rare metabolic disease phenylketonuria (PKU). Furthermore, it's safety for young children, pregnant or nursing women, and those with liver or kidney disease has not been established. The DLPA form is less likely to raise blood pressure than the straight L-form.

If you are concerned about the possible side effects of using amino acids, consider the following: In her experience with using amino acids for depression, Dr. Patricia Slagle has stated that "in all the years I have been treating depression with amino acids, I have never had to discontinue the treatment because of side effects. I have, at most, had to modify the tyrosine and phenylalanine usage in cases of preexisting high blood pressure."

Remember to never modify or stop taking any drugs prescribed by your physician without his or her supervision.

Overall Guidelines for Successful Amino Acid Therapy

Amino acids should not be given to young children, elderly people or anyone taking MAO antidepressant drugs without professional consultation and guidance. If you are taking MAO inhibitor drugs, taking tyrosine can raise your blood pressure. Because of these issues, I recommend that you find a doctor who is willing to work with you, and that you supplement your amino acids with vitamin B6. Vitamin B6 boosts the body's amino acids and may allow for smaller amounts of tryptophan and tyrosine to be used. A vitamin B6 deficiency causes a large amount of available tryptophan to be converted to by-products, which may actually cause the level of serotonin to decline. (Vitamin B6 is part of the core protocol for depression, so you'll be taking it anyway.)

When you begin to take amino acids, you may feel worse at first. Be assured that this is a common reaction. Patricia Slagle, M.D., has found that a combination of amino acids and vitamins is usually effective within the first two weeks of use. She points out that most antidepressant medication takes four to six weeks to take effect.

To be most effective, amino acids should be taken at the proper time each day. Take amino acids on an empty stomach, and do not take with any protein food such as milk. Taking amino acids with a small amount of fruit juice (to enhance its transportation) is also suggested.

Some Last Thoughts on Amino Acid Therapy for Depression

5-HTP, L-tyrosine and DLPA are considered the most effective amino acids for treating depression. These three amino acids act as precursors to brain amine synthesis. When the body suffers from a lack of any of these amines or neurotransmitters, a drop in mood can occur and depression can result. Research done at MIT has concluded that tyrosine and tryptophan play a profound role in determining the rate at which four crucial brain chemicals are produced. These amino acids directly affect blood levels of these mood-controlling neurotransmitters, especially serotonin. Because of this, amino acids may be a key piece to solving your depression puzzle.

Amino acid therapy works by creating an excess of amino acids, which, in turn, forces the body to create increased amounts of neurotransmitters like serotonin. As a result, feelings of depression or melancholy are directly impacted. Technically, drugs like Prozac are designed to accomplish the same goal, which is to elevate these brain chemicals, thereby creating a feeling of well being, but they come with side effects not experienced with amino acid therapy.

CHAPTER 20

Herbal Prozac: St. John's Wort and Ginkgo Biloba

Herbs and plants are medical jewels gracing the woods, fields and lanes, which few eyes see and few minds understand. Through this want of observation and knowledge the world suffers immense loss.

LINNAEUS

A STUDY PUBLISHED in a 1999 edition of *Psychosomatic Medicine* states:

> A number of herbs and dietary supplements have demonstrable effects on mood, memory and insomnia. There is a significant amount of evidence supporting the use of *Hypericum perforatum* (St. John's wort) for depression and *Ginkgo biloba* for dementia. Results of randomized, controlled trials also support the use of kava for anxiety and valerian for insomnia.

Hallelujah, the medical community has finally acknowledged the medicinal value of herbs! It has been estimated that as much as 75 percent of the population of this planet utilizes herbal medicines. What is not commonly known is that this widespread use of herbs is not limited to poor or backward nations. Almost half of all medical doctors in France and Germany use herbal therapy as part of their healing strategies.

Throughout this book, I too have suggested herbal treatments as key pieces in solving the depression puzzle because I feel that they are safer and come with less side effects, while being as good or better than traditional treatments. These natural approaches also tend to treat the body as a whole, and they see the interconnectedness of different body systems. In fact, one can learn a lot about the herbal approach to depression puzzle-solving by investigating ancient views of depression.

Ancient Views of Depression

Depression in ancient Gaelic medicine was traditionally linked to a disruption of the melancholic humor. The Chinese have viewed depression as a disturbance in the *chi* or natural energy of the human body and would recommend chi-moving herbs to treat mood disorders. The crown Chakra, which is associated with the pineal gland, would be targeted for treatment with herbs like gotu kola and nutmeg. In Ayurvedic medicine, which is derived from two Indian words—*ayur,* or life, and *veda,* or knowledge—depression is seen as a disruption of the state of vata and kapha, which directly affects the nerves. Eastern medicine considers any emotional disorder as a sign of any number of physical diseases and commonly employs herbs to treat depressive illness. Invariably, all ancient practices view the body as part of an integrated whole. In light of this approach, depression—like other diseases—is considered a disruption in the ideal balance of all body systems that collectively create something we call "health."

While all of this may sound a bit like hocus pocus, there is much to be gleaned from centuries of herbal medicine. If you carefully interpret what may sound like bizarre or primitive views, you often find a sound scientific truth behind ancient perceptions. For example, depression can be a disruption of a delicate biochemical balance that is affected by a number of body systems. If one of these systems gets out of whack, in domino fashion, several others are thrown off. Botanical medicines offer a complete array of biocompounds that are designed to work with the body instead of against it. Because they are natural, they come with far less side effects than synthetically engineered drugs. One of the best plant extracts for the treatment of mood slumps is called St. John's wort.

St. John's Wort: An Introduction

When it comes to herbal medicine, European practitioners have left American doctors in the dust. St. John's wort is the most widely prescribed treatment for depression in Germany. Over sixty-six million daily doses of St. John's wort were prescribed in Germany for depression, nervousness and anxiety in 1992—a statistic that tells us great numbers of people want to feel happier without using prescription antidepressants. St. John's wort is prescribed four times as often as Prozac in Germany and adds up to a total of approximately $72 million in sales. Moreover, its costs are covered by German insurance companies. In America, Prozac is the third leading prescription drug, whereas in Germany, it has earned less than a 2 percent market share.

I recently read a magazine ad for Prozac that said, "Remember, Prozac is a prescription drug, and it isn't right for everyone." What I want to know then is, why is everyone on it? Interestingly, Prozac's patent runs out in 2003, at which time some people predict that Prozac will become available in an over-the-counter form.

In light of the glut of Prozac and other antidepressant drugs we consume in this country, one might assume we have no need for an herbal antidepressant, but nothing could be farther than the truth. American sales of St. John's wort have increased by over 11,000 percent in the last few years. Why? Because as Peter Breggin says in his book *Toxic Psychiatry,* antidepressant drug effects are short lived, with little or no evidence for sustained relief, and their hazards are considerable. In addition, a great many people who try antidepressant drugs stay depressed. Furthermore, their doctors rarely take the time to question them about their lives, eating habits, relationships or other factors to get at the root of the problem.

I received a letter from one woman who was having a terrible time with unexplained depression. She asked her doctor about the impact of nutrients on mood. He replied, "Nutrition and supplements have no bearing on your emotional status." She writes, "I was angry, embarrassed and humiliated . . . I went to see another internist who tried to put me on Prozac five minutes into the visit." She goes on to say that she wishes "the medical community would get back to the basics, lose their egos, listen to their patients and educate themselves about natural simple alternatives." One of the best of these is St. John's wort.

How Does St. John's Wort Work?

St. John's wort, also known as *Hypericum perforatum*, is a plant that sports yellow flowers and commonly grows in the wild. A compound called hypericin is the primary bioactive chemical in St. John's wort. The exact way that St. John's wort produces its antidepressive effect is still unknown, but it seems likely that it works through a number of different pathways simultaneously.

One of the earliest studies with hypericin in 1984 indicated that it may reduce the amount of a brain enzyme called monoamine oxidase (MAO). MAO breaks down serotonin, so when its levels go down, serotonin goes up. (It should be noted, though, that many experts think that this most likely is not the method by which the herb functions) St. John's wort may also work to actually block an enzyme called catecholo-methyltransferase, which works to break down brain chemicals.

Other studies have suggested that St. John's wort may act as a selective serotonin re-uptake inhibitor (SSRI) much like Prozac and other SSRIs. St. John's wort may also block the re-uptake of two other mood-regulating neurotransmitters, dopamine and norepinephrine.

The herb's action on the immune system may also impact mood. St. John's wort suppresses cytokine release, particularly interleukin-6. Cytokines are immune system molecules that also act as messengers between the central nervous system and the hypothalamus, adrenal gland and pituitary gland. Consider the fact that interleukin-6 may be one of the compounds that over-stimulates these glands, leading to elevated levels of cortisol. (Remember that this is the hormone released when we become stressed.) St. John's wort causes a significant suppression of inter-leukin-6, which acts to stabilize these overactive glands, thereby producing a tranquilizing and mood-boosting effect.

Research on St. John's Wort

Scores of studies have been published on St. John's wort. In fact, over 5,000 test subjects have participated in trials designed to eval-uate St. John's wort for depression. An analysis of over twenty stud-ies published in a recent article of the *British Medical Journal* sug-gest that St. John's wort may be just as good as antidepressant drugs, with none of the side effects associated with synthetic med-icines. The studies used 300–1,000 mg of St. John's wort extract taken daily for a period of four to eight weeks. Twice as many patients taking the extract responded positively to treatment than did the placebo group. The researchers used the Hamilton Depression Scale, a standard diagnostic tool used to assess the severity of depression. For example, sleep disturbances or feelings of sadness are assigned a numerical value and are added up. A lower score represents a decrease in depression. This overview published in the August 3, 1996, *British Medical Journal,* found that the herb may be useful in cases of mild to moderate depression.

In another current study, 105 patients were given either 900 mg of St. John's wort standardized to a 0.3 percent hypericin content each day or a placebo. After four weeks, they were tested with the Hamilton Scale to measure the status of their depression and found that 67 percent of the St. John's wort group decreased depression by over 50 percent. Skeptic or not, these are impressive statistics for a plant extract. (I might add here that the mood boosting properties of St. John's wort aren't limited to human beings. An article in *Time Magazine* talked about using the herb for depressed dogs and was aptly titled "St. Bernard's Wort"!)

St. John's Wort Challenges Prescription Antidepressants

Clearly, research suggests that St. John's wort may afford a depressed person comparable depression relief and far fewer side effects than with conventional antidepressant drugs. Eight studies compared St. John's wort extract to standard antidepressants, such as imipramine, bromazepam and maprotiline. The dose of extract was 500 to 900 mg daily. Interestingly, more patients responded favorably to St. John's wort (63.9 percent) than the antidepressants (58.5 percent). Of equal importance is that only 19.8 percent of the St. John's wort patients experienced side effects, while 52.8 percent of the patients on the conventional drugs reported adverse effects.

Similar results were obtained with severely depressed patients in another study published in a 1997 issue of *Pharmacopsychiatry*. St. John's wort extract (600 mg, three times daily) was given to 209 patients for six weeks, while the control group received imipramine (50 mg, three times daily). In short, St. John's wort offers relief from depression with far fewer side effects than do available drugs. And dozens of other studies confirm these test results.

The National Institute of Mental Health and St. John's Wort

Several doctors have recognized the profound value of this herb and have candidly admitted that St. John's wort extract may not be just an herbal alternative but also a viable option when considering effective approaches to depression. In fact, because of its excellent safety profile and tolerability, St. John's wort can be the first line of treatment for depression, according to some experts.

In fact, the National Institute of Mental Health (NIMH), in collaboration with the NIH Office of Alternative Medicine (OAM), has launched a three year, 4.3 million dollar study to investigate this herb and whether it has any value for people with clinical depression. It will be headed by Dr. Jonathan Davidson, a psychiatrist at Duke University Medical Center. Davidson has said that he is impressed that so many mainstream medical school researchers have contacted him to express their interest in participating. This study will involve 336 patients with major depression (as defined by the *Diagnostic and Statistical Manual of Mental Disorders,* Fourth Edition). Patients will be assigned randomly to one of three treatments for an eight-week trial. One-third of the participants will receive a uniform dose (900 mg daily) of St. John's wort, another third will receive placebo, and the other will be given a selective serotonin re-uptake inhibitor (SSRI), commonly prescribed for depression. Keep in mind that because pharmaceutical companies cannot obtain patents on herbs, studies such as this one must be funded by the government or other public or private sources.

St. John's Wort and Weight

In addition, St. John's wort may prove useful in treating obesity. I have found that when you are working with brain amines like serotonin, hunger is almost always affected. You probably know that Phen-Fen artificially raised serotonin levels to discourage eating. Perhaps St. John's wort works similarly, although there are currently no scientific studies on the effectiveness of St. John's wort for weight-related problems. However, if you think that you overeat because you're depressed, consider taking St. John's wort to boost your mood while you diet.

Other Medicinal Properties of St. John's Wort

In addition to its benefits for depression, St. John's wort has been shown to be useful in treating seasonal affective disorder (SAD) and sleep disorders. It also has significant antiviral activity (against HIV, herpes, hepatitis C, influenza and Epstein-Barr) and can promote tissue healing in wounds due to its antibacterial action.

Hypericin not only works to raise mood, it is also under investigation as a possible treatment for AIDS. Apparently, hypericin can bind to cell membranes and cross-links virus proteins. In so doing, it scrambles the infective properties of viruses and can render them sterile. It also exerts a similar action on cancerous tumors, especially when potentiated by light or laser.

Dosage and Safe Use of St. John's Wort

Typical doses of St. John's wort for depression range from 300 to 900 mg daily of 0.3 percent hypericin product. The Core Protocol suggests taking 300 mg three times daily. Some new St. John's wort products are now available and have been standardized to 3–5 percent hyperforin.

Possible side effects based on European data include dry mouth, dizziness, gastrointestinal symptoms, increased sensitivity of sunlight, fatigue and confusion. Be aware that these effects are rare and usually mild. Safety issues concerning St. John's wort usually focus on the possibility of photosensitization, although it has only been reported in one person and in animal studies. If you are concerned, wear protective clothing or sunscreens while taking it.

If you find that the herb makes it difficult for you to sleep, combine it with passion flower or kava kava root. Remember that serotonin-raising compounds can cause insomnia. Adding B vitamins and 5-HTP can also help. Don't take the herb after six in the evening if insomnia continues to be a problem.

A CAUTIONARY NOTE

Anyone taking an antidepressant should not go off of it or alter its dosage unless supervised by a physician. Taking St. John's wort with prescription medications is not advised. If you want to get off drugs and try natural alternatives, talk to your doctor and work out a sensible plan. St. John's wort is also used for the treatment of attention deficit disorders, seasonal affective disorder, sleep disorders and lack of sexual desire (which means that it could lift the spirits of not only the one who takes it, but of their spouse as well). Talk to your doctor before taking St. John's wort if you are over age sixty-five, currently taking any medications, or if you suffer from headaches, heart disease, or liver or kidney dysfunction. The herb is not recommended for children under twelve years of age, pregnant women or nursing mothers. If you use this herb, it may take up to six weeks for its antidepressive effects to take effect. St. John's wort as a sole treatment is not recommended for serious or major episodes of depression.

The Last Word on the Wort

Hyla Cass, M.D., a board-certified psychiatrist and author of *St. John's Wort: Nature's Blues Buster,* has stated that for a fraction of the cost, St. John's wort can be as effective as prescription antidepressants without the numerous side effects that often accompany these drugs. Unfortunately, American physicians are slow to acknowledge St. John's wort as a legitimate treatment for depression. It has been suggested that if studies continue the way they're going, St. John's wort will eventually enter the medical mainstream.

Ginkgo and Mood

Ginkgo biloba is another herb that has enjoyed tremendous popularity over the last decade as a memory booster and possible treatment for Alzheimer's disease. It works to increase blood flow to brain cells, thereby improving mental functions. Its benefit for depressed individuals has only recently emerged, especially regarding the notion held by some experts that depression is a condition of brain cell understimulation.

Ginkgo's antidepressant action may hinge on its ability to boost brain cell oxygenation by enhancing blood flow. In several studies using ginkgo for memory problems, researchers observed an unexpected benefit. Many of their test subjects who took the herb experienced an elevation of mood. A French double-blind study found that 166 patients with mental disorders significantly improved with ginkgo therapy. Other studies that have noted the positive effect of ginkgo on mood have prompted scientists to look into the possibility of using ginkgo to treat depression.

A study published in 1990 evaluated the use of ginkgo in sixty patients suffering from depressive symptoms in combination with some form of dementia. The results showed significant improvements among those given ginkgo extract instead of the placebo. Another study followed forty depressed individuals over the age of fifty who had not responded successfully to antidepressant therapies. Those who took ginkgo showed a drop in Hamilton Depression Scale scores of 50 percent, while the placebo group showed only a 10 percent improvement.

How Does Ginkgo Improve Emotional and Mental States?

A report published in 1994 studied levels of serotonin receptors in rats of various ages. When older rats were given ginkgo supplementation, the number of serotonin-binding sites increased, but this effect was not seen in younger rats. The researchers speculated that ginkgo may work to prevent the loss of serotonin receptors due to aging.

Obviously, the fewer serotonin receptors you have, the harder it is to sustain mood. In fact, with less receptor cells, you would need even more serotonin to create the desired effect on mood. However, ginkgo takes a new therapeutic approach to mood elevation. Instead of raising the level of serotonin like Prozac does, it enhances the brain's ability to respond to serotonin, making the process more efficient, especially in older individuals. Of course, more studies are needed to confirm this effect; however, I believe that ginkgo's long list of credentials as a brain booster makes it a natural choice for depressive illness.

Dosage: The typical dose of ginkgo is 40 mg taken three times daily. Use a 50:1 extract standardized to contain 24 percent ginkgo flavonone glycosides and 6 percent terpene lactones. It usually takes from two to eight weeks for full benefits. Ginkgo leaf extract appears to be quite safe. In over 9,000 people who were given standard ginkgo formulations in double-blind studies, the most common side effect was mild stomach discomfort, which only occurred in less than 0.2 percent of test subjects. Headaches and dizziness were also reported. You should not combine ginkgo with blood-thinning drugs. There is also a remote possibility that combining ginkgo with natural blood thinners such as garlic, phosphatidyl serine and high doses of vitamin E may also cause abnormal bleeding. The safety of ginkgo for young children, pregnant or nursing women, and those with liver or kidney disease has not been established.

Caution: Never stop taking an antidepressant or any other drug without the supervision of your doctor. Mixing certain herbs and drugs can also be undesirable, so please proceed only under your doctor's care.

Guidelines for Purchasing and Using Herbal Medicines

When considering the purchase of an herbal supplement, probably the most important thing to do is look for guaranteed-potency herb products with standardized active ingredients. Virtually every clinical study performed on herbs or other natural substances works with active ingredients that must be taken in certain dosages to achieve desired results. Not every herbal product guarantees potency; as a result, you could waste your money and time, not to mention the fact that if you neglect to see any desired result, you may conclude that natural therapies are worthless. However, as herbal treatments become more mainstream, you are more likely to find more high-quality products. For this reason, it is vitally important that we, as consumers, take advantage of the most current and reliable data concerning botanical medicine.

At the moment, herbs are still classified as food or food addi-

Practical Tips for Selecting Herbal Supplements

- Choose herbal forms that are the most effective for the particular problem. Herbs can come in extracts, tinctures, dry capsulized powders, and even ointments and creams. Also, look for the percentage of active ingredient, if possible. New delivery systems such as sublingual drops or creams may provide even better assimilation.
- Do your homework on the specific herb you have chosen to take. Find out which form of the herb works best for your ailment rather than taking every herb that is mentioned for a particular ailment.
- Give children only a fraction of the adult dose depending on their age, and don't give children under the age of two any supplement unless you check with your physician. Children six to twelve typically can take one fourth of the adult dose, and children twelve to eighteen, three fourths of the adult dose. Exact dosages vary from herb to herb.
- Herbs are designed to work with the body and usually require consistent use over a long period of time to achieve the desired results.
- If you are prone to allergies, pregnant, nursing or taking other drugs, check with your doctor before using herbs.
- Keep all herbs out of the reach of children. If large amounts of an herb are ingested by your child, contact poison control immediately. There are also herbal guides that list toxic dosages and their effects.
- Knowing whether an herb should be used orally or topically is particularly important, as well as recommended concentrations of the herb. Wild yam, for example, is better when absorbed through the skin rather than taken orally, and tea tree oil should only be applied topically.
- Purchase herbs from reliable sources that you know are pure. Look for standardized products with guaranteed potency. Also, try to use products that come from ecologically aware companies that are sympathetic to the environment.

Practical Tips for Selecting Herbal Supplements (cont.)

- Read the contraindications of certain herbs and make sure that you do not have a condition that may cause an unwanted reaction. Also, be careful about mixing drugs and herbs. Even common herbs (ginseng) and over-the-counter drugs like aspirin can have negative interactive effects. The *Lancet* recently published a review of unwanted herb-drug interactions that can be viewed for free online at their website (www.thelancet.com).
- Take dosages that are recommended, and don't assume more is always better. Time, not quantity, brings positive results.

tives; therefore, manufacturing companies cannot by law list any of their therapeutic applications or recommended dosages on bottle labels. For this reason, consumer awareness is crucial. Herb users need to use herbs judiciously, and never assume that just because a substance is natural, it can be randomly taken in excess amounts. The ephedra scare is a good example of what happens when people consume herbal preparations without adequate knowledge of what they are taking. And while herbs are usually classified as foods, they must be used judiciously—in the proper amounts and for the right ailments. They are still agents that produce chemical reactions in the body. See the accompanying sidebar, which provides guidelines that may help you in your determination of which supplemental products to buy and use.

Are Herbs Safe?

Andrew Weil, M.D., a widely respected and popular physician who promotes the best of both conventional and natural medicine, states, "For every prescription I write for a pharmaceutical drug, I give out forty or fifty for botanical remedies. In almost 10 years of prescribing in that way, I have not yet seen a serious adverse reaction in any patient taking a medicinal plant." Statistics support his views: From 1983 to 1992, there were no deaths from herbs, three from all dietary supplements (from contaminated tryptophan and iron poisoning), 320 from over-the-counter drugs, 9,000 from food-born illness, and 100,000 from prescription drugs. Herbs can be very safe if used as directed. However, the notion of "more is better" should not be applied to herb usage—many herbs have dangerous side effects when taken in dosages higher than recommended.

CHAPTER 21

Acupuncture and Other Holistic Treatments for Depression

IT MAY SOUND somewhat archaic to some, but using needles to treat a variety of diseases is nothing new. Acupuncture is finally beginning to get respect among health care practitioners who can't deny studies that support its use as a therapeutic agent. And when it comes to mood, a new report shows that acupuncture may reduce or eliminate symptoms of depression. A new pilot study by Dr. John Allen at the University of Arizona in Tucson, in collaboration with Tucson acupuncturist Rosa Schnyer, suggests that acupuncture may be at least as effective as drug therapy in the treatment of depression. This double-blind study, sponsored by the National Institutes of Health Office of Alternative Medicine, compared the symptoms of major depression in three groups of women. For an eight-week period, the first group of women received specific acupuncture treatments designed to target depression. The second group experienced acupuncture for symptoms not associated with depression. The last group was put on a waiting list. Neither the women nor the acupuncturist knew what group they belonged to.

After eight weeks, the women who had received specific acupuncture treatment for depression were significantly less depressed than the other women. Interestingly, the authors of the study also discovered that a slight trend in depression reduction occurred in the women who were given other acupuncture treatments as well.

Still many wonder, why explore treatments like acupuncture for depression when there are so many other effective treatments? A large-scale study sponsored by Harvard Medical School and published in the *New England Journal of Medicine* reported that depression was among the most frequently reported conditions, and one of the top five conditions for which people were more likely to seek alternative treatments (with or without established treatments) over established treatments alone. Acupuncture was one of the alternative treatments mentioned. (I must add that if you believe the crux of this book—that physical disorders are often at the heart of depression—acupuncture offers another bonus. It can also be used to treat a variety of specific physical symptoms.)

We may not know all the reasons why some people choose alternative treatments for their depression, but there is a growing body of evidence that shows the effectiveness of some of these treatments on mood, without sufferers ever having to take a prescription drug. This chapter will explain what some of these other treatments are and how they work. As you puzzle-solve your depression, consider experimenting with some of these treatments. You may even find the solution to your depression in this section alone—without having to take any herbs or supplements. Let's begin by taking a closer look at acupuncture.

How Does Acupuncture Work?

According to Chinese medical tradition, acupuncture works by altering or channeling the flow of energy along various meridians of the body. Chinese data suggests that when particular points along meridians are stimulated, certain effects occur. Acupuncture involves contacting specific acupoints by the insertion of very fine needles. It is designed to augment the flow of chi or energy, to restore the proper balance to affected organs. Knowing what points to target is essential. The careful evaluation of a person's symptoms is necessary and is based on physical markers combined with a series of questions.

While acupuncture needles appear somewhat terrifying, their insertion is rapid and is usually painless. These needles come in a variety of sizes designed for specific insertion points. Blood is usually not drawn if the needles are inserted correctly. Acupuncture has the distinct ability to either stimulate or calm certain nerves. Combining the use of natural supplements with acupuncture can create an effective treatment plan for depression. Of course, finding a qualified acupuncturist is vital and can determine whether the treatment succeeds or fails.

Magnet Therapy and Depression

In addition to acupuncture, the use of magnets as therapeutic agents has gained popularity over the last few years. In fact, magnet mania created all sorts of healing claims not supported by evidence from double-blind studies. Usually, treatment consisted of portable magnets of mild intensity placed on painful areas in order to influence electromagnetic fields and mask pain.

Recently, however, powerful magnets were applied to the heads of test subjects to treat depressive illness and the results were rather surprising. Transcranial magnetic stimulation is the technical term for this innovative and rather fascinating new treatment for serious depression. Emory University researchers report that more than half of the patients treated improved with no serious side effects. These magnets actually stimulated a specific region of the brain (the left-front portion), which is thought to be underactive in some people suffering from mood disorders. The treatment only lasted five minutes during which time the electromagnet creates an electric current through the brain, causing brain cells to fire connections that stimulates the production of brain chemicals like serotonin.

To date, magnet therapy has only been used for people with severe depression. But although the treatment is still considered experimental, the results are encouraging and once again support the idea that sleepy brain cells can cause us to feel depressed. Waking up nerve connections in certain people results in a marked improvement in mood. The long-term effects of magnet therapy are unknown at this point in time, however. In must also be stressed that playing around with strong electromagnetic fields can be dangerous. Like electroconvulsive therapy (ECT), using magnets to alter brain function must only be done under the supervision of a physician.

Using Aromatherapy to Fight the Blues

Someone once said that "an unexpected whiff of a familiar but long forgotten scent can precipitate a rush of emotions fraught with nostalgia, delirious joy or unspeakable sorrow with more impact than any other form of recollection." In fact, anyone who has been emotionally touched by a scent cannot deny the power of aromas on the mind. Anything from pumpkin spice to grandpa's aftershave can change mood, enhance memory or intensify emotion. In fact, using scents to effect changes in the body (aromatherapy) has been done for centuries. Fragrant oils were used by the ancient Egyptians and Israelites, not to mention a number of Eastern cultures.

Dr. Rene-Maurice Gattefosse, who is considered the father of modern aromatherapy, has stated, "Doctors and chemists will be surprised at the wide range of odoriferous substances which may be used medicinally." Aromatic oils are commonly used in foods, perfumes and medicines. We have also seen a sudden rise in aromatherapy products such as candles and room sprays. So what exactly are essential aromatic oils?

Essential oils are concentrated aromatics that easily evaporate when exposed to air. They are extracted from fragrant plants and are partially soluble in water. Because heat, light and moisture compromise the integrity of these oils, they are kept in dark, air-tight bottles. There are a great number of scents available—anything from rosemary to peppermint to cedar wood can be used to make an essential oil.

Each scent also has a different effect on the body. Various studies conducted to assess the psychological effects of essential oils conclude they can either stimulate or calm the nervous system. Doctors at the University of Milan demonstrated the benefit of certain aromatic essences in relieving states of anxiety and depression. At the University of Milan, depressed patients were treated with a combination of sandalwood, orange, verbena, lemon and jasmine oils. For anxiety, bergamot, neroli, cypress, orange leaf, lime and marjoram oils were applied. The citrus oils they used for depression were indigenous to Italy and included bergamot, lemon and orange. These oils were successful in helping to dissipate the depressive illness in the test subjects. (Furthermore, patchouli oil has been employed for a number of years in European mental institutions to prevent psychotic reactions, and bergamot is traditionally used to treat manic depression.)

The validity of aromatherapy has spawned considerable controversy in conventional medical circles. Most of us are aware of the bad reputation that "sniffing something" has received over the past few years. By the same token, if inhaling caustic substances can produce bad neurological symptoms, then the opposite must also be true. In fact, the therapeutic mechanics of aromatherapy have been ascribed to the effect fragrance has on the limbic system.

HOW DOES AROMATHERAPY WORK?

According to Dr. Claudia S. Miller, M.D., M.S., there are three physical routes through both the nose and the mouth in which substances can affect, stimulate or even cross over into brain tissue. The limbic system of the brain is where mood, short-term memory, long-term memory and smells are stored. Specific smells can act as stimuli, consequently, certain neurotransmitters are released. Some smells, particularly chemical oils, can produce extremely unpleasant emotional reactions. By contrast, natural oils can evoke a variety of pleasant sensations, including the elevation of mood. The use of herbals in the form of essentials oils for their aromatic value can greatly benefit anyone who is depressed. Using these oils in combination with massage therapy, in baths, facial saunas, and steamers can help to boost mood. A combination of chamomile, jasmine and bergamot is recommended for depression. Other essences that are considered mood elevators include lavender, clary sage, melissa and tiferet-lifetree. (One way to use fragrant oil is to place the drops on a brown sugar cube.)

Meditation, Stress and Mood Control

Another therapy garnering considerable attention over the last few years is meditation. The ancient pharaoh Akhenaton once said, "Contemplate thy powers, contemplate thy wants and thy connections; so shalt thou discover the duties of life and be directed in all thy ways." By now, we've established the fact that if you're suffering from depressive illness, you probably need to alter your brain biochemistry to get well, but this approach is not a cure-all for low moods. The fact remains that if you don't learn to get in touch with your inner self through exercises like regular meditation, the day-to-day stressors of life will continually wreak havoc on your mood and outlook. As long as you are inundated with stress without any productive way to diffuse it, your brain chemistry will continue to be undermined.

The little voice that goes with us everywhere and continually provides us with an hour to hour analysis of who we are and how we're doing can either make or break us. If you choose to focus on despair, suffering, injustice and tragedy, you will see little else. The ways in which we deal with everyday stressors are excellent examples of how negative factors can limit our capacity to feel happy.

Today, the market for stress relievers is tremendous. Stress reduction has become a multi-million dollar industry. For those of us who fight depression, stress is an even bigger problem. Who among us isn't dealing with significant stress? Trying to eliminate stress is usually nothing more than an exercise in futility. Hence, we need to learn to manage stress. Hans Selye views stress as a positive thing. He states, "Stress is the spice of life. Complete freedom from stress is death."

Dealing with troubles is the great common denominator all of us share. It can bind us together as we struggle to work through it, or it can crush us. In all probability, if I asked you why you might be feeling depressed you might answer, "my boss is so demanding," or "I hate my marriage," or "my children are driving me crazy," or "there's never enough money," or "I have to take care of my mother who has Alzheimer's disease" and so forth. The truth is that the underbelly of our lives reveals multiple hardships. In the midst of our sorrows and stress, however, it can make us stronger and more capable. In order to turn stress into something positive, however, we must learn how to deal with it—especially if we discourage easily. Studies of stress tell us that if you're under too much of it without a positive outlet, your serotonin levels can become depleted. Hence, you can become profoundly dismal and downcast.

MEDITATION HELPS SMOOTH OUR "RUFFLED FEATHERS"

A report published in the May/June 1998 issue of the *American Journal of Health Promotion* showed the transcendental meditation (TM) to be two to four times more effective in reducing stress and anxiety than other stress reduction programs. This type of meditation creates a state of restful consciousness that stimulates the body's inner mechanisms to eliminate accumulated stress and fatigue. Many of us are wary of meditation and feel uncomfortable when we attempt it, but remember that Samuel Coleridge said that "there is one art of which man should master, the art of reflection." Most Americans neglect to set aside time for reflection.

Unfortunately, like so many ancient healing practices, meditation has often been overlooked as a marvelous healing tool. Being able to meditate teaches us how to access deeper states of consciousness. Meditation can effectively block out the negative thought patterns that threaten to destroy us during a bout with depression. Meditation also helps us connect with our subcon-

312 • SOLVING THE DEPRESSION PUZZLE

scious minds. In so doing, feelings of spiritual awareness and tranquility can be produced.

When you meditate, marked changes in your physiology occur, as well as a clarification of thought processes. Dr. Benson, in his book *The Relaxation Response,* demonstrates that meditation can normalize blood pressure, lower pulse rate, decrease the levels of stress hormones in the blood and produce changes in brain wave patterns.

The American Journal of Health Promotion reports that TM or transcendental meditation can even result in the decreased use of cigarettes, alcohol and drugs. Another study recently published in the American Heart Association's journal *Hypertension* reported that the TM technique lowered high blood pressure better than exercise and diet modifications. In fact, transcendental meditation was shown to produce blood pressure reductions equal to those commonly found with medication. And because depression involves so many body systems, regular meditation can be of great benefit, especially when it comes to neutralizing the kind of thinking that is generated in a depressed mind.

THOUGHTS CAN AFFECT BRAIN NEUROTRANSMITTERS

How can meditation have such a profound affect on the body and, in particular, the brain? Scientific research supports the notion that thoughts and feelings affect neurotransmitter production. Habitually engaging in negative, anxious or hostile thoughts can alter the chemical makeup of the brain resulting in behavioral changes—and potentially, changes in the health of the body. A steady diet of undesirable images and thoughts determines how we feel and what choices we make. It is for this very reason that the impact of violence and sex in movies and television on America's youth is of such concern. Our minds are impressionable and vulnerable to manipulation. Regarding the many detrimental influences we are exposed to, meditation works like damage control for the mind.

HOW TO MEDITATE

Now that we know what meditation can do for our health, we can tackle a second issue—how exactly do you meditate effectively? There are several ways to meditate, and they are all designed to achieve the same end. You can focus on a symbolic sound (mantra), a single image (mandala), or you may choose to become acutely aware of the rhythmic patterns of your own breathing. Any of these methods produce a deep, calm, restful, trance-like state that frees the mind from anxiety and confusion.

Concerning the value of meditation, Bernie Seigel, M.D., in his

---

The Power of Meditation

While we've talked specifically about the transcendental type, meditation can take all sorts of forms. It can include yoga with deep breathing and biofeedback training. All of these types of meditation have one thing in common—they achieve a state of "mindfulness." Mindfulness refers to the ability to let the mind go completely blank by not concentrating on one particular thought. Ironically, while the term "mindlessness" may seem more appropriate, the "fullness" concept refers to the notion that while the mind is full, it is not focused on any one subject. Whether it be this way or another, we should all practice meditation regularly for fifteen to twenty minutes every morning or at least ten to fifteen minutes twice a day. Meditation is a real medicine for the cumulative effects of stress and depression. Don't expect overnight results. Just keep at it and practice regularly.

Research has shown the positive effects of meditation will last two to three weeks after one stops; however, if you do stop, the benefits will eventually cease. Remember, so often we look outside of ourselves for the answers to personal dilemmas. Learning to meditate can sharpen the tools we all have to heal from within.

314 • SOLVING THE DEPRESSION PUZZLE

book, *Love, Medicine and Miracles,* says, "I know of no other single activity that by itself can produce such a great improvement in the quality of life." It's too bad that something as beneficial as meditation is not routinely taught in our culture. Again, ancient civilizations were more knowledgeable about the value of healing therapies than we have managed to be in our highly educated, high-tech society.

In fact, the practice of meditation can actually alter brain function, endocrine function and boost the immune system, three areas that are intimately linked with depressive illness. If you're feeling down, you think in a certain way. In other words, you get into the habit of continually bombarding your mind with pessimistic ideas. Meditation can help stop negative thought patterns.

Keep in mind that learning how to effectively meditate will not be easy. Most of us have to fight our strong resistance to clearing our minds of conscious thought. The Buddhist reference to the untrained mind as a "drunken monkey stung by a bee" probably applies to most of us. Because true meditation is difficult to cultivate, make sure you use it only as a supplement to other therapies for depression. There are several good instructional books available on meditation. Most of them suggest sitting down, with your back straight either on the floor or on a chair. Your aim will be to direct all your attention to a particular object such as a flickering flame. Your mind will inevitably wander from your chosen object, and so you will redirect your attention back. You will have to do this over and over again until you master the ability to prohibit distractive thoughts from entering your consciousness. Transcendental meditation can be achieved by sitting in a comfortable chair for fifteen to twenty minutes twice a day with your eyes closed.

Biofeedback

As mentioned in the previous section, meditation can take all forms, including yoga and biofeedback. When it comes to the value of biofeedback, the words of Bhagavad Gita seem appropriate: "The mind is restless, turbulent, obstinate and very strong. To subdue it is more difficult than controlling the wind, but it is possible by constant practice and attachment. He who strives by right means is assured of success." Technically speaking, biofeedback is based on the idea that if we become aware of certain body functions, we can learn to control those functions through thought patterns.

Biofeedback uses instruments designed to monitor brain waves, blood pressure, skin temperature, heart rate, etc. Through a feedback system, a person can learn to alter involuntary functions they normally have no control over. For example, the ability to warm the hands, relieve muscle tension and lower blood pressure are just a few actions that can be accomplished through biofeedback.

Recent work with epileptics who have been taught to ward off seizures through this type of self-awareness suggests that other neurological disorders may benefit from biofeedback. Some studies suggest that depressed people, like some epileptics, have a particular brain wave pattern.

The electrical activity of the brain can be classified into four types. Each correlates to a particular brain function and state of mental awareness:

Alpha Waves. These waves create a calming and clearing effect on the mind that is usually accompanied by a state of relaxation. Alpha waves can lead to more heightened levels of awareness.

Beta Waves. These waves comprise the normal working rhythm of the brain. When beta waves become faster, they reflect activity and stimuli. States of relaxation produce very little beta wave activity.

Delta Waves. Delta waves are typical of sleep states but can be produced in some people when they are stimulated by a new idea or concept.

Theta Waves. Periods of meditation or creativity are usually characterized by theta waves.

CAN DEPRESSION CREATE ITS OWN BRAIN WAVE?

Margaret Ayers, director of research at the Los Angeles-based Biofeedback and Advanced Therapy Institute, found (after five years of research) that primary depression without a manic component can manifest itself in a specific brain wave pattern. This pattern is characterized by slow waves and high voltage. Ayer's objective was to use biofeedback to change the biochemical profile of the brain, thereby affecting a psychological change. The notion of changing brain wave pattern to change emotional behavior has not been successfully done in the past. The concept, however, seems scientifically sound.

In 1975, scientists discovered that brain waves recorded while epileptics slept revealed a distinct pattern of disorganized sleep and a tendency for motor twitching. Scientists reduced the number of seizures suffered by these epileptics by using biofeedback. Additional results were also noted. These unexpected effects of biofeedback treatment included increased concentration and energy, less aches and pains, and a feeling of mental invigoration. In studying these findings, Ayers theorized that symptoms of depression could also be affected in the same way. She was able to fine-tune the voltages of a biofeedback unit and enlisted the help of three depressed individuals to test her theories.

What she discovered through their EEGs was that their waking brain wave patterns resembled those of the epileptics. By using biofeedback techniques that train the patient to suppress unfavorable wave patterns, she was able to cause behavioral changes in depressed patients. In other words, these depressed individuals succeeded in inhibiting the specific brain wave pattern that was associated with their depression. At the same time, they were able to produce another brain wave that suppressed feelings of depression.

All of these patients were examined by a clinical psychologist who was not told that they had undergone prior biofeedback treatment. The findings were consistent. The depression had been reversed. Like the epileptics, these patients also became more mentally alert and experienced a surge in energy. Their mysterious aches and pains were greatly reduced or totally disappeared. As long as the brain wave pattern was changed, the beneficial results persisted.

WHAT ARE THE MECHANICS OF BIOFEEDBACK?

How does biofeedback for depression work? Surface electrodes are placed on the scalp using a one-inch strip that runs from ear to ear. These electrodes are hooked to a neuroanalyzer unit that is connected to a polygraph. The polygraph records filtered brain wave patterns on paper.

In this type of biofeedback, the patient experiences an EEG feedback. In other words, they are given positive rewards for achieving certain brain wave patterns in the form of an orange light, a certain digital number, or a beeping tone. These rewards serve as positive reinforcements for the elimination of negative frequency bands; whereas, a red light indicates that the desired brain wave alteration is not occurring. The treatment then gets progressively harder in order to train the individual to control his or her physiology to a greater degree and with more success.

Ayers believes that when the brain becomes depressed, it gets into a rut and doesn't know how to correct itself. Based on this theory, she believes biofeedback can be tremendously beneficial in guiding the brain back to its normal state. Remember our discussion on the sleepy brain syndrome and how it can cause a depressed mind set? The brain, in its attempt to achieve a homeostasis or normal biochemical balance, is capable of producing high-frequency brain waves that suppress slow wave activity. Her findings show that biofeedback teaches the brain to accomplish this in such a way that both brain wave patterns eventually disappear.

The normal period of time required for depression-oriented biofeedback therapy is between two and three months. Typically, a biofeedback training program consists of ten hour-long sessions every week or so. Even though the time intervals may be a drawback, study results are promising.

Research findings imply that biofeedback may provide a noninvasive treatment for depression, designed to implement a learned brain wave pattern. It may offer a viable, long-term alternative for people who suffer from depression. Like so many other therapies, the possible benefits of biofeedback for depression should be investigated further. (Biofeedback has also been successfully used for treating migraine headaches, hypertension, Raynaud's disease and stress-related disorders.)

ADDED BENEFITS OF BIOFEEDBACK IN TREATING DEPRESSION

Elmer E. Green, Ph.D., who founded the Biofeedback and Psychophysiology Center of the Menninger Foundation, believes that any chronic condition with a psychosomatic link can be treated with biofeedback. In fact, he thinks that one of the most promising aspects of biofeedback for depressed people is the realization that one can control what are considered involuntary processes of the body. This creates feelings of empowerment and self-mastery crucial for anyone who is depressed because depression snatches away control.

Many insurance companies now cover biofeedback and some hospitals have practitioners trained in the technique. This fact alone has elevated the status of biofeedback within the medical community. People who respond best to biofeedback are those tenacious individuals with a strong ability to visualize.

Controlled Breathing

Another therapy related to meditation is controlled breathing. Like biofeedback, our human bodies contain built-in healing powers that often remain inaccessible due to simple ignorance. Breathing can be used for much more than the oxygenation of our cells. Breathing exercises can be surprisingly effective at dispelling mental fatigue, relaxing the nervous system, and creating a sense of tranquility. The change in perspective that is possible with this therapy is also important, especially considering a statement by Ralph Waldo Emerson: "Everything intercepts us from ourselves."

Controlled breathing can help you understand and deal with these constant interceptions.

How do you learn controlled breathing? Every day at the same time (or when you feel particularly unable to cope), concentrate on your breathing. Put everything else out of your mind and become acutely conscious of each and every breath you take. Once you are practiced in the method, you should be able to see the positive effects it can have on the psyche.

Several yoga books contain good breathing exercises; however, any good system works on the same principles:

• Position the tongue against the back of the teeth throughout the exercise. Begin by first exhaling completely through the mouth. Making a hissing sound can help to expedite a complete expulsion of air in a slow, controlled manner.
• Next, begin to inhale through your nose with your mouth closed while you are counting to five in your head. Now, hold your breath for approximately six to seven seconds. Begin to exhale slowly through your mouth, making the same hissing sound and count to seven in your mind.
• At this point, take another breath and repeat the same sequence of events. You can do this three to four times.

Controlled breathing exercises like this one have a wonderful tranquilizing effect and should be done on a daily basis or as many times as your feel you need to. Some experts recommend using breathing techniques to dissipate not only stress or anxiety, but also insomnia. They can also be combined with controlled, isolated body stretches for added relaxation. This type of therapy is called progressive relaxation and is discussed later in the chapter.

When you're depressed, you know how difficult it can be to do something as simple as relax. Manipulating your breathing can exert a strong influence on the mind, the body and your mood by creating true relaxation. In many respects, breathing exercises are nothing more than another form of meditation. Controlled breathing is easy enough to do and incorporate into your life. I have personally found that it is an invaluable way to dispel the kind of mounting stress we often encounter in the work place or in dealing with family stressors. Keep in mind that it is normal to feel a little lightheaded when you first start.

Massage Therapy

There are also more "hands-on" therapies that can have a positive effect on mood. For instance, manipulating or rubbing the deep tissues of our musculature can stimulate us both physically and mentally. Applying touch or pressure to certain muscle groups through massage therapy can help to restore function and surprisingly, actually improve mental outlook.

There are several schools of massage from the Chinese and Japanese to the Swedish. American Indians also used massage to achieve relaxation through what involved vigorously brushing the body rather than actually rubbing it. Why do so many cultures make use of massage techniques for healing?

The value of massage therapy stems from idea that when nerves are stimulated through muscle groups, feelings of well being and exhilaration can be created. Being touched is a basic human need and some experts believe that when you're depressed, that need is intensified. The combination of physical and mental benefits hold great healing potential.

In addition, massage therapy with scented oils takes advantage of both muscle manipulation and aromatherapy as well. The penetrability and aroma of essential oils enhances the benefits of massage. Continual rubbing and kneading of not only the neck, shoulders and back, but also the forehead, face, chin, top of the hands, chest, and feet stimulates nerve endings and boosts peripheral circulation. Scalp massages are also excellent for both physical and mental fatigue and can help to restore feelings of energy and elevate moods.

Remember that feeling anxious, restless, irritable, sleepless or sad can all be reflected in your posture and the state of your muscles. Tense individuals who suffer from chronic stiff necks know all about this phenomenon. We unconsciously manifest our emotional states in our musculature, much more so than most of us imagine. Regular massage can help to counteract the negative effects daily stressors inflict on the body and the mind.

TYPES OF MASSAGE

Taoist masters used a massage system called chi lei jong that concentrated on massaging the abdomen. It is particularly good for redirecting blood flow and stimulating the lymphatic system. It can even be self-administered. Swedish massage, which usually comprises several basic strokes applied to soft body tissues, can tranquilize the nervous system. This vigorous form of massage stimulates circulation and can relieve tension. It is also used to help individuals cope with various emotional problems. Some experts even believe that the very act of massage can help bring emotions to the surface.

Keep in mind, however, that the effects of any massage or aromatherapy are only temporary. But if these therapies are done on a regular basis, their cumulative benefits are far from minimal. If you can't afford regular massages, invest in a good, electrical massage unit. New models include shiatsu massage units that apply deep rhythmic massage and high intensity pulsating units. When you feel overly tense or just need to unwind and clear your mind, use one of these machines for ten minutes. The effects are quite refreshing. Your attitude will invariably improve after a treatment.

If you want professional massage treatments, ask around and make an appointment with a skilled and reputable therapist. The money involved for massage therapy is well worth the rewards and is really quite inexpensive considering what we willingly spend on manicures, perms, golf, etc.

Progressive Relaxation

Another technique, progressive relaxation, can be done on your own. This particular technique produces a feeling of relaxation and is especially good for treating insomnia and anxiety. The exercises are easy and are based on a simple procedure of alternating between a state of tension and relaxation in the muscles. Initially, you contract a muscle as hard as you can for a period of two seconds, after which you totally relax that muscle. You repeat this exercise for another muscle and then another, until your entire body falls into a state of sublime relaxation.

• Lie on your back and take two deep, controlled breaths before you start.
• The usual sequence starts with the muscles of the face and neck, and then progresses to the upper arms, chest and back. The process is repeated for the abdomen, buttocks, thighs, calves and feet.
• You may want to start by clenching your teeth and squeezing your eyes and work down to making tight fists, and pulling your stomach muscles in toward your spinal column. Make sure that you go completely limp after each contraction.
• If you need to, repeat the whole process again and then lie perfectly still with your eyes closed.
• Listen to the natural rhythm of your breathing and concentrate on remaining free from tension of any kind. Some experts recommend taping sequential step by step instructions for this exercise on a cassette and playing it right after you get into bed. This particular method can be used at work or during the day if you feel yourself tensing up. Progressive relaxation can be done in any position.

You can train yourself to become very adept at progressive relaxation. The idea behind this technique is that by contrasting the differences between tension and relaxation, the latter is intensified. In time, you'll have the order in which you tense and relax muscle groups down, and the exercise will become automatic. The following muscle groups are recommended:

Forehead: wrinkle your forehead and relax.
Mouth: open your mouth as wide as it goes and then bite down and

clench your jaw (not too tightly or you could damage your jaw joint), then relax.

Shoulders: lift your shoulders to your ears, hold, then relax.

Chest: inhale and fill your lungs completely, hold for three seconds then slowly exhale and relax.

Arms: clench your fists and contract your arm muscles hard, then relax.

Stomach: bulge your stomach out as far as it can go then pull in it as hard as you can, then relax.

Back: arch your spine as high as you can get it of the floor, hold it, then relax.

Hips and upper legs: rock your knees and exert pressure on your heels, digging them into the floor, then relax.

Lower legs and feet: lightly curl your toes while you extend your legs out, lift them off the floor, keeping them stiff, then relax.

Progressive relaxation is a marvelous way to unwind and combat the kind of stress and anxiety that would hurt our ability to feel tranquil or sleep well. Remember to concentrate solely on what's happening with each muscle group and don't let your mind wander. Part of the reason that so many of us can't relax or get to sleep is that we let our attention slip into dismal thought patterns that directly impact a number of biological systems with negative input.

Music Therapy

While few physicians ever refer to the medicinal effects of music, Martin Luther put it well when he said, "Music is the art of the prophets, the only art that can calm the agitations of the soul." Unquestionably, what we hear can profoundly affect the state of our nervous system—ask anyone who lives with a teenager. Music directly and indirectly impacts the subconscious mind. It can create feelings of tension and irritability or peace and serenity. Ancient cultures have known the power of music from the beginning of time. They have used drum rhythms and ritual sound repetitions to prompt sensations of ecstacy, mysticism, sexual excitement and hypnotic states.

Likewise, noises that commonly fill our environment can subconsciously determine our state of mind. Although most of us are unaware of background noises, they can subtly color the way we see things and how we feel. I've found that sometimes my subconscious perception of TV dialogue playing in another room can make me feel jumpy and progressively tense, especially if I'm trying to read or work at the computer.

If you suffer from depression, it's important to choose specific kinds of sound for your environment. Certain sound effects seem to be universally beneficial. Slow moving classical music, soft jazz, and certain nature sounds like rain falling usually serve to calm and pacify. On the other hand, strong, rhythmic drum beats, high-pitched noises, and loud fast moving music can grate on the nerves and create emotional disturbance.

MUSIC AND PHYSIOLOGY

In hospitals, relaxing music has been shown to actually decrease blood pressure in coronary patients. The most effective type of music seems to have a tempo of around seventy to eighty beats per minute, which is almost the same as the average pulse rate. In depressive illness, music therapy serves to break down walls that can make you feel isolated from the rest of the world. It can, in some cases, enable a depressed individual to feel more talkative or even outgoing. Music has been used more extensively over the last few years to not only stimulate the nervous system of depressed people, but to draw people with autism and schizophrenia out of their private worlds.

Be aware that just because a selection of music seems calm and mellow doesn't mean it's desirable for melancholia. Some kinds of music are intrinsically sad and evoke like feelings. For example, the soundtrack to the movie *Schindler's List* is full of profound sorrow and should probably be avoided if you're fighting depression. By contrast, lively Baroque instrumental music has been used in Europe for its ability to create a sensation of well-being and mood elevation. Some studies have shown that when you listen to this type of music, your heartbeat will eventually synchronize itself with the musical beat and relaxation will occur.

Other kinds of desirable music and sounds include gentle ballads, classical guitar, spiritual compositions, waves pounding, bird songs and night crickets. Put on uplifting music when you get up and when you come home. Don't underestimate its power to make your heart glad.

CHAPTER 22

"Exercise" the Demons of Depression

The body is a test tube. You have to put in exactly the right ingredients to get the best reaction out of it.

JACK YOUNGBLOOD

UNDERSTANDABLY, IF YOU'RE suffering from depression, exercising is the last thing you feel like doing. In fact, depression has been described by some experts as a state of high energy turned inward. For this reason, trying to suppress or deny depression can only make it worse. But if you think of depression as a form of negative energy, then the prospects of transforming that energy into movement can make more sense. Some experts believe that depression can be a form of anger turned outside in. Marjorie Brooks, Ph.D., of Jefferson Medical College in Philadelphia says, "Low-grade depression is found more often in women than in men. Some women may feel powerless at times, but instead of getting mad, they get depressed. As a result, they may constantly feel tired or have a chronic headachy feeling." How can individuals prevent the depressive effects of anger and frustration?

Releasing these feelings through exercise is highly recommended by many experts for its variety of beneficial effects. More and more research supports the fact that exercise is a powerful therapy against mood fluctuations. Robert S. Brown, Ph.D., M.D., and his colleagues at the University of Virginia have utilized a number of different physical activities to snap their patients out of depressive states. They believe, to some extent, that the dramatic lack of movement that is so typical of a depressed person may in itself aggravate further depression.

Most depressed people are consumed with unhappy thoughts. Some, so much so that they can actually become physically incapacitated. Some doctors believe that if you sit around too long, you may develop what is called a primary movement disorder, which always makes depression worse. Numerous studies have proven that if you break out of lethargic behavior and force yourself to move, a more positive self-image will emerge. Even minor, low-impact exercise like walking around the block can create significant beneficial psychological changes. I believe that exercise is an essential piece in the depression puzzle and should be implemented along with any other treatments you choose to take.

Exercise: No Better Antidepressant

Andrew Weil, M.D., claims that he knows of no better method to relieve the symptoms of depression than aerobic exercise in the form of thirty minutes of continuous activity at least five days a week. A recent article in the *Journal of the American Psychological Association* explores the beneficial relationship between exercise and mental health. The authors reviewed the results of various studies in which exercise was used as a treatment for individuals with clinically diagnosed psychiatric disorders, including depression. They found that regular exercise was a viable, cost-effective therapy for mild to moderate depression and may even be useful in the comprehensive treatment of more severe episodes. Of particular interest was the fact that although aerobic exercise is usually recommended as the most effective, more passive forms of exercise such as weight lifting and strength training were just as effective in treating depression. The study concluded that exercise is underused as a treatment, in spite of the fact that numerous studies consistently describe it

Physical Activity: The Depression Workout

Dr. John Greist, who has written a paper entitled "Running Out of Depression," conducted a study of twenty-eight depressed patients and found that those patients who regularly ran controlled their depression much better than those who were treated with psychotherapy. Even if you can only get out three days a week, the emotional benefits of regular exercise cannot be overstated.

as a powerful and effective tool for treating many diseases and disorders, both physical an psychological.

Unfortunately, very few physicians will recommend exercise as part of a treatment plan for their depressed patients. And often, unless their physicians advise them to exercise, depressed patients will not do it as a part of their treatment.

You Can't Feel Sad and Exercise at the Same Time

What's even more encouraging is that it's almost impossible to feel sad while your exercising. Dr. Russ Jaffe, Director of the Princeton Brain Bio Center, maintains that "recent onset depression is hard to sustain with low-impact aerobic exercise." He goes on to suggest swimming, bicycling, cross-country skiing, and even brisk walks followed by both a warm shower and a cold shower. He claims that these activities are powerful weapons against depressive illness. The psychological benefits of regular exercise cannot be overemphasized. Exercise can help you get in tune with your body and its needs. While you're exercising, your mind's activity is stimulated, leading to increased meditation and ultimately the unraveling of some of the problems you might be facing. In addition, exercise naturally does what drugs try to accomplish—it elevates certain brain amines that make us feel happier.

Exercise Stimulates the Release of Mood-Boosting Brain Chemicals

Most of us know about brain chemicals called endorphins. Studies show that after a certain amount of sustained exercise, brain endorphins are released that create feelings of invigoration and well-being. Marathon runners have often described the euphoric states of consciousness they experience after running.

It is also true that aerobic exercise causes norepinephrine to be released in brain cells, and by now, you should be well aware of the fact that depression can be caused by a deficiency of norepinephrine. In many depressed individuals, norepinephrine—measured by detecting a substance called MHPG—is lacking. Exercising causes MHPG levels to rise. As a result of this elevated level of norepinephrine, depression can be reversed and synaptic transmission in the brain stimulated. Exercise acts as a wake up call to your brain cells. Even more, the phenomenon lasts even after you stop exercising.

In addition, when you jog or walk briskly, serotonin is also increased. Positron emission scans have revealed that during exercise, the right part of the brain is activated, resulting in fantasizing, uncluttered thinking and a state of mental awareness. In addition to this, serotonin, which determines mood, rises. As a result, you feel happier.

Learning to walk briskly every day or to jog at a moderate pace not only eases the blues, it provides a whole host of physical benefits as well. Vigorous regular exercise can also help relieve insomnia, poor appetite, irritability and anxiety—symptoms that usually accompany depression, and it is very inexpensive.

Two of the basic requirements for a healthy and happy life are fresh air and exercise, to which the benefit of sunlight exposure is also added. Even on an overcast day, the light intensity is around 10,000 lux. For anyone suffering from a seasonal affective disorder, exercising for thirty minutes outdoors is the equivalent of a daily session of light therapy.

Exercise Guidelines for Beating the Blues

Decide now to make regular exercise a part of your life. Below are some guidelines to help you not get started on and stick with a regular exercise regimen:

• Above all, start slow and take it easy.
• Before you begin to exercise, remember that no fitness program can be truly successful if you don't utilize the powers of the mind as well as the body. You must want to be healthy. Desire is everything.
• Brisk walking is especially good. Let's face it, the aging process itself can be depressing and walking is a great anti-aging defense. If you walk briskly for at least fifteen to thirty minutes a day, you can expect to feel a considerable mental and physical lift. If you can find a walking companion, that's great, but walking alone can also have its benefits. Walk a dog, walk where and when it's safe, and walk consistently.
• Choose the time of the day that feels most natural and affords you the best opportunity for success. Don't pick four in the morning to go running unless you're a morning person. Exercising after work or before dinner is just as good.
• Establish a routine. Do it for your physical, emotional and spiritual well being.
• Exercising with a companion is recommended, as is using music to enhance your workout. It can energize your body and elevate your mood. Scientific studies have proven that music makes exercise more enjoyable and easier to accomplish.
• You might want to incorporate jogging or walking as your main mode of transportation. During your lunch break, get out of the office and eat lunch outside. Walk around the block before you return to work.
• You should also check with your physician to make sure that exercising is a good idea for your particular situation.

Body Motion Oxygenates Brain Cells

Exercising can also raise the oxygen level of your cells, which can directly impact how much physical and mental energy you generate. When you breathe deeply, you expedite the removal of carbon dioxide and other waste from your body systems. Remember that during states of depression, regional blood flow to brain tissue is usually decreased. Exercising can help to reverse this. Remember our discussion on the benefits of using SAMe for depression? There is some speculation that the faulty removal of toxins from brain cells can bring on episodes of depression. Exercising helps to facilitate the removal of harmful waste material from the brain.

As we talked about earlier, some experts have claimed that it is virtually impossible to sustain a mental state of anger, depression or anxiety during and right after vigorous exercise. Some studies have shown that jogging for thirty minutes three times a week can be as effective or even more so than psychotherapy sessions. In fact, Rita Moreno, a well-known performer, has passionately related how regular exercise literally saved her from an emotional crisis she experienced during menopause.

Moreover, if you've felt low for an extended period of time, you may suffer from a myriad of aches and pains. Regular exercise can help to alleviate stiff muscles and joints and can boost the digestive system so elimination is more efficient. When you exercise, you sleep better, breathe easier, and think clearer.

In addition, a recent study reported that exercise was the only way to counteract the weakening effects that depression has on the immune system. Periods of depression can actually lower lymphocyte levels (immune cells that fight off disease). The study found that those depressed individuals who exercised were able to better protect their immune system defenses.

By now, it should be clearly understood that exercise can be a powerful antidote to depression. Vigorous workouts can not only initiate chemical reactions that elevate mood, they can also give you a sense of purpose and control that helps to dispel gloom. To the person who suffers from depression, exercise should be viewed as nothing short of life saving.

CHAPTER 23

Spiritual Healing

For he will command His angels concerning you to guard you in all your ways; they will lift you up in their hands, so that you will not strike your foot against a stone.

PSALMS 91: 11–12

IN THIS CHAPTER we will return to a topic discussed in the beginning of the book—the role of spiritual healing in treating depression. I firmly believe that if healing is our top priority, we must do much more than just work with the body. I recently read about a veterinarian and a taxidermist who decided to share a shop in a small town. The sign in their front window read, "Either way you get your dog back." There's a lesson behind their humorous motto, however—about the body and the spirit. We don't want to just get the body back, but unless we work to heal the spirit, we are really nothing more than walking corpses. In our effort to regain our health, we must look at ourselves as whole and unique individuals made of flesh and spirit.

Once again, I hate to seem like a doctor basher, but the medical community rarely inquires about the spiritual state of its patients. Recent Gallup polls tell us that the American people need to reclaim a spiritual dimension when dealing with sickness or terminal illness. George Gallup writes, "Doctors are not as a group nonreligious or irreligious—however, they could be much more aware of the spiritual connection in treating their patients."

Sadly, the notion of physician as healer and advisor has been lost. People take more time to discuss the pros and cons of a car purchase with a salesman than to go over their health concerns with a doctor. Conversation is usually minimal and limited to the brief description of a few symptoms. By contrast, natural health practitioners ask detailed questions concerning every aspect of a person's life, including the spiritual. I firmly believe that no matter what therapy we use or promote, or regardless of how impressive any natural supplement is, we must address the whole person when dealing with any illness. By whole I mean the body and the spirit. This is not only true of disorders like depression, but of any disease we may encounter.

The spiritual aspect of healing is such an important piece of the depression puzzle that it can't be overlooked. In fact, this piece affects not only the depressed individual, but also those around them. We've talked about various therapies for depression, but we haven't addressed the needs of someone who lives with a depressed individual. Let's talk about those who struggle to understand the depression of a loved one.

Dealing with Depression Requires Charity

For those of us who are not depressed but love someone who is, much is required. Let me be perfectly candid here. When it comes to dealing with a depressed individual, friends and loved ones often feel frustration and anger, and they may feel like throwing in the towel. I've discovered that while charity implies long suffering, patience and bearing each others burdens, it sometimes means intervening to change what can become a vicious and self-defeating cycle. Practically speaking, I have learned that listening with a spirit of love can prevent overreacting to the vocabulary of depression. Yes, we need to be aware of warning signs, but we also have to learn to cope with the language and demeanor of depression by tapping into spiritual sources of strength, and seeing it for what it really is.

Depression Numbs Our Spiritual Receptors

A depressed person often turns away from God and faith. Much the way serotonin receptors can malfunction in the brain, our ability to feel the healing power of God may also become impaired. If you love a depressed person who has lost their faith, becoming defensive or feeling responsible for how they feel is not productive. If someone you love says, "I wish I were dead," understanding that statement for what it is, rather than taking it personally, is so important. Often we blame ourselves if someone around us feels sad. You may think, "If I had raised her right, she wouldn't feel so hopeless," or "What kind of a wife am I if my husband is always battling depression?" No good comes from these thoughts so get rid of them. Becoming defensive, anxious, sad or depressed as a reaction to a depressed individual only aggravates the situation. You can't fight negativity with negativity. Stay upbeat and happy—for your own sake. Show your loved one how sweet life can be through your example.

Patience and Empathy Are Vital

Of course, trying to rouse feelings of gratitude or spirituality in someone who feels depressed rarely succeeds, especially when we resort to lecturing. I have found that preaching to a depressed person serves no good purpose. I believe that this is where patience combined with a proactive attitude comes in. Stop asking them why they are sad or how they got so low. Moreover, don't continually ask a depressed family member or friend how they are. In other words, don't keep pulling up the plant to see how the roots are doing. I'm afraid I'm guilty of this with my own children. Let me also say that I still struggle to tame my tongue, because I know that a listening ear would be more therapeutic than delving, probing and assessing.

Living with a depressed person can be one of the most depressing of all things, but it is a part of the journey, another challenge that we face as mortals trying to make our way through the maze of this world. Believing in the power of unconditional love and the power of the human touch, while being willing to wait as the healing process takes place, is what it's all about. We must realize that like so many of life's other trials, depression can be overcome. Moreover, we can be better for having experienced it, as it contributes to the person we eventually become—one who is more aware of the fragility of the human spirit, more empathetic with the plight of humans and stronger in will.

Faith Precedes the Miracle

When Gustauv Courbet, a famous painter from 19th century Paris, was asked why he never painted an angel, he replied, "Because I have never seen one." Unfortunately, like Courbet, we are generally a skeptical, cynical, "seeing is believing" oriented society. It matters little what religious denomination you may belong to. Nurturing faith, no matter how weak it may be or what you have faith in, is still important to complete healing. My sister has a quote carved in wood that is strategically placed over her mantle. It reads: "Credendum vides," or "Believing is seeing." In essence, the opposite of the skeptical approach to life. In other words, it is only when we believe or exert faith that certain truths are made known to us—truths we may not have otherwise seen, truths we need to know about ourselves or a particular individual. I am one who believes that none of us will ever feel totally whole or content until we acknowledge the presence of a power greater than ourselves.

Carl Jung, in treating people with psychological disorders, wrote, "It is safe to say that every one of them fell ill because he had lost that which the living religions of every age have given to their followers, and none of them have been really healed who did not regain his religious outlook." Depression snuffs out faith, hope and charity, and causes a kind of amnesia to settle over our minds so that we forget how to feel the sustaining spirit of God.

Even atheists and agnostics agree that the probability of any one of us being here on this planet as the result of a cosmic accident is infinitely small. Lewis Thomas tells us that you'd think the mere fact that we exist would keep all of us in a continual state of wonder. Sadly, as humans, we don't react that way. We routinely become accustomed to miraculous events—like our own existence, for example.

I firmly believe that hopelessness is not of God, and that being depressed is like walking through the valley of death. Even something as difficult as depression gives us a chance to learn more about God. Even the experience of depression has divine possibilities for us. Each and every experience and affliction we endure can add to our character. Albert Schweitzer once said, "We gather strength from sadness and from pain. Each time we die we learn to live again."

Draw on the Powers of Heaven

Certainly many of us have been gravely disappointed in our lives. Unquestionably, many of us are confused—troubled by issues of sexuality, intimacy, moral values, marital discord, difficult children and other equally important matters. But when we close the door on our spiritual selves, we can quickly become unfamiliar with the language of the spirit. And by so doing, we deprive ourselves of a marvelous healing dimension. Thank goodness drawing on the powers of heaven is not the taboo subject it was a few years ago. As we enter a new millennia, great segments of our population are openly admitting their need for spiritual nourishment. The soul has been badly neglected and even abused by our societal focus on money, power and gain. Within academic and intellectual circles, the worth and value of nurturing our spiritual selves has typically been mocked. In our efforts to employ the scientific method to validate anything and everything, we have forgotten the ultimate healing power of spiritual medicine.

Our hesitance to include supernatural help when healing disease ultimately does us a disservice, especially when we are formulating treatment plans for depression. Why are we afraid to encourage the incorporation of spiritual aids as a way to get well? Is it because people will think we're a bit eccentric, naive, or maybe even a little strange? Lily Tomlin has jokingly said, "Why is it when we talk to God we are said to be praying, and when God talks to us we're said to be schizophrenic?"

The Very Real Therapeutic Power of Prayer

If you're battling with depression, you need to trust more in powers unseen to fortify yourself. In so doing, you can truly discover who you really are and your immeasurable worth as a living soul. Goethe said, "As soon as you trust yourself you will know how to live." Trust your ability to get in tune with your spiritual self. Trust that there is a loving God who is aware of your struggles. Ask for help and expect to receive it. Man was created that he might have joy, not despair.

If you decide to try natural therapies, remember that unlike the scientific community, you can expect miracles. C.S. Lewis expresses it beautifully, "By miracles, we don't mean contradictions to nature. We mean that left to her own resources, she could never produce them." I would strongly suggest that all of us employ the power of prayer to facilitate the miracle of wellness.

When you rise in the morning, pray. Express gratitude for life and thanks for the opportunity to be alive and then let our Creator know what your specific needs are. Ask in faith, believing that you are loved and that your life is precious. One study called "The Efficacy of Prayer" by Plant J. Collipp, M.D., suggested that prayer can indeed have real value in the treatment of disease. Dr. Collipp states, "Among the plethora of modern drugs and the increasing ingenuity of our surgeons, it seems inappropriate that our medical literature contains so few studies on our oldest and, who knows, perhaps most successful form of therapy [prayer]."

If you don't have any spiritual roots, cultivate some. Seek out whatever you believe God to be and learn to have faith. Never underestimate the power of love that helps us break out of our obsessive preoccupation with ourselves. Know that your life has meaning. Believing that we're here as the result of a random cosmic coincidence is the most depressing thing I've ever heard. It's not true.

Throughout the pages of this book, we've explored the notion of getting in touch with our inner selves through meditation, relaxation etc., but prayer is very rarely suggested in most self-help literature. How many of us have tried to cultivate a personal rapport with our Creator? Even the current religious resurgence many of us see all around us can never take the place of the private cultivation of a deep and intimate relationship with God. All the psychoanalysis and all the antidepressants in the world can never heal us so completely. Seeing the world through spiritual eyes can reveal a very different picture. Albert Pike said that, "Life is what we make it and the world is what we make it. The eyes of the cheerful and of the melancholy man are fixed upon the same creation, but very different are the aspects which it bears to them."

CHAPTER 24

The Game Plan: An Overview

Happiness is nothing more than good health and a bad memory.
UNKNOWN

ANN LANDERS ONCE said, "One out of four people in this country is mentally imbalanced. Think of your three closest friends—if they seem okay, then you're the one." If you're the one suffering from depression, stop and rethink your dilemma. If we've learned anything from our discussion, it's that depression is a complex disease impacted by nutritional, environmental and lifestyle factors. A notion which also tells us that depression can be cured by altering those same factors.

The simple truth is that everything we put in our mouths, as well as where and how we live, determines our health and happiness to a great degree. Look around; take an inventory of how you live. Investigate your lifestyle and make some changes. Each factor is a clue, a piece in the puzzle of your depression. And each piece you find and place in this puzzle moves you closer to a solution. Hopefully, this book has helped you begin the puzzle-solving process, leading to possible solutions to overcoming your depressed state.

Inevitably, however, certain questions remain. For example, does a depressed mood initiate changes in our biochemistry or is the opposite true? Perhaps the answer is that the cause and effect of mood and chemistry should be viewed as a continuous loop of biological reactions. Everything we do, from gulping down a cup of coffee with a doughnut to working in a poorly lit office, can profoundly affect the delicate biochemical balance of our bodies and change our mood. Likewise, any changes in mood can initiate biochemical changes and other physical problems. And each factor reinforces the others, perpetuating the mood disorder.

This cycle of depression can be discouraging, but don't despair. This book has the keys you need to fight back. For instance, by now you know what depression is, what causes depression and what methods are available to reverse depression. This knowledge is the first step toward empowerment. Now it is up to you to apply what you know and to keep trying. And while we continue to explore the mysteries of the human body and its psyche, remember that there already exists a substantial body of evidence that natural medicine can effectively treat many forms of depression. That in itself is cause to celebrate.

I also know that many of you may still not know where to begin, despite the knowledge that has been presented to you so far in this book, and that's okay. This chapter is meant to be a jumping off point, a place to start. The important thing is to start now. Don't put it off. You can begin recovery today—this very minute.

Become Proactive

The first piece of advice I want to give you is to be proactive. There is much we can do to scare the goblins of depression away and get on with the business of living. Helen Keller, who had every reason to curl up and die, put it beautifully when she said, "The world is very full of suffering, it is also full of the overcoming of it." Based on my own experience, I believe that even in the midst of your darkest winter, you can find your invincible summer. Let's be frank—its not going to be easy, but it is certainly attainable.

You now have the necessary tools, and they are at your disposal. You can and will feel happy again. Believe that. When you learn how to rebalance your body, contentment will not be something that you have to feverishly pursue. It will just happen. All of us need to have a reason to get up in the morning. To find that reason, we must live by a life map, or a set of guiding principles. If you've lost your map, form another one and always remember that when we nourish and care for our body and spirit, they have a miraculous ability to heal themselves.

Even though the majority of this book has been dedicated to explaining the biological reasons behind depression, recovering from depression should be about more than just following the core protocol and supplementary guidelines for treating depression. As discussed in the chapters on alternative therapies and spiritual healing, nutritional and herbal therapies may be more effective when combined with other lifestyle changes and additional activities—like exercise, prayer and meditation. In fact, breaking the habits of depression may require more than just dietary changes and supplements. The following guidelines can help you become proactive by pointing you to habits that foster contentment and happiness. However, these should in no way take the place of other treatments described in the book or drugs prescribed by your doctor.

The Antidepression Day-Plan

• A light box may be beneficial when you first wake up, or flood your environment with sunlight or artificial light. Turn on a lot of lights if it's dark. If not, open your curtains to get more sunlight.
• Eat breakfast and take your core protocol supplements for depression as well as other nutrients for other individual disorders. Try to eat a meal that contains some protein (meat, eggs, peanut butter, nuts, cheese, cottage cheese). Balance out your breakfast protein with fresh fruit and whole grain bread or cereal. Avoid caffeine, refined sugars and white flour.

344 • SOLVING THE DEPRESSION PUZZLE

How to Create an Antidepressive Environment

• Fill your home with wonderful aromas by using light bulb rings, diffusers, steamers and essential fragrant oils. Coming home to a house filled with the smell of cinnamon can go a long way in promoting a sense of tranquility and well-being.
• Get a pet.
• Get plenty of sunlight. If sunlight is not available, obtain adequate sources of strong artificial light. Install a skylight or invest in a light box.
• If the news depresses you, cancel your newspaper subscription and/or watch a video or read instead of tuning in to the evening news.
• Play uplifting music that makes you feel optimistic.
• Surround yourself with plenty of green plants, fresh flowers and other growing things. Cultivate a garden.

• If you can exercise outdoors, do it during the daytime (especially when it is sunny). If not, move on a treadmill, with a video, etc. Always focus on breathing deeply, which will more fully oxygenate your blood.
• If you feel yourself slipping, call a friend or a support telephone line and chat for a few minutes.
• Play uplifting music throughout the day.
• Pray or meditate. (Show gratitude for specifics in your life and ask for support to do the things you have planned for the day.)
• Seek out humor throughout the day. See a funny movie, read a humorous book, or listen to a comedy tape or CD. Clip out funny cartoons and post them.

Beneficial Habits To Form and Maintain

• Consistently cultivate a spiritual philosophy that is centered around a loving God.

• Get a weekly massage using essential oils or use a home unit.

• Get outside and exercise on a regular basis. If the weather is disagreeable, make sure you exercise indoors. Invest in a piece of equipment you are most likely to use. Treadmills are usually very good and are utilized more than fancy contraptions that cost a fortune.

• Practice controlled breathing exercises at least once a day, and use progressive relaxation techniques to unwind.

• Pray often.

• Take a hot bath with aromatic oils every night thirty minutes before retiring.

• Take your nutritional supplements every day, and watch your diet.

• Use daily meditation or breathing exercises to center your life and prevent mood swings.

• When you get home from work, pop in a soothing and mood-elevating tape or CD (e.g., Baroque strings, Mozart, Kenny G).

Afterword

IF THERE EXISTS in medical annals a disease that proves the delicate interconnecting relationships between the mind and the body, it's depression. The most stunning discovery to emerge from studying research compiled for this book is the fact that even the most minor disruption of brain chemistry can result in feelings of anxiety, depression and discontentment. Moreover, what causes these disruptions can be something as insignificant as a lack of sunlight or a subtle enzyme dysfunction in the brain.

Serotonin levels in the brain, which are extremely important in the determination of mood, can be decreased by a number of seemingly unrelated factors. Amazingly, these factors can react to each other making the question of what-causes-what-first very difficult to determine. There can be no question, however, that everything we do, what we eat, the chemicals we are exposed to, stressors and our genetic code can affect brain biochemistry and alter mood.

It is in the area of naturopathy, which emphasizes the links among diet, environment and mental health, that the safest potential cures for depression are found. The secret lies in finding out for yourself—being empowered. Remember that even if your depression is the result of a sad event, nutritional and emotional support can only serve to help you better cope with your situation.

It is also vital to understand when approaching a complex disease like depression with natural medicine that there are individual differences in the way each person will respond to the treatments discussed in this book. What is essential is to locate a doctor or health care practitioner who is willing to work with natural therapies and tailor them to fit your needs.

You might be asking yourself, if natural treatments for depression are as safe and effective as presented in this book, why don't more physicians recommend them? Generally speaking, the med-

348 • SOLVING THE DEPRESSION PUZZLE

ical profession uses therapies that are familiar and considered standard treatments. Unfortunately, it takes a great deal of effort to test out alternative treatments and doctors usually don't take the time to investigate any out-of-the-ordinary therapies. As a result, if a doctor is not familiar with a particular treatment program, he or she will probably be skeptical.

The way we view diseases like depression will undergo dramatic changes during the twenty-first century. Doctors will be forced to educate themselves about the profound role that nutrition plays in the healing process. Inevitably, the physician of the future will concentrate on the prevention of disease and its treatment through diet and natural supplementation. Thomas Edison foresaw this rebirth of natural medicine when he predicted, "The doctor of the future will give no medicine but will interest the patient in the care of the human frame, in diet, and in the cause and prevention of disease."

Resolve now to do everything you can to prevent depression from cheating you of your life. There are no "miracle cures," but miracles happen every day. Don't stand in the way of your own healing miracle. Jack Paar hit it on the head when he said, "Looking back my life seems like one long obstacle race, with me as its chief obstacle." If you want to get well, arm yourself with knowledge, put it into practice, and never give up. Remove the word "impossible" from your vocabulary and utilize the information you have been given. Keep in mind that what were once described as bogus remedies for all sorts of diseases are today's scientifically supported solutions. And never forget that none of us will ever know complete health until we recognize ourselves as spiritual beings clothed in physical bodies.

Bibliography

Abraham, G. "Management of fibromyalgia: Rationale for the use of magnesium and malic acid." *Journal of Nutritional Medicine.* 3 (1992): 49–59.

Adler, Jack. "Biofeedback: Physiological means to treat depression." *Let's Live.* (1982 January): 28–31.

Ahokas, A. et al. "Role of estradiol in puerperal psychosis." *Psychopharmacology.* 147, number 1 (1999 November): 108–110.

"Altered serotonin metabolism in depressed patients with Parkinson's disease." *Neurology.* 34: 642–646.

American Journal of Psychiatry. 156 (1999): 1149–1158.

American Psychiatric Association. Drug Facts and Comparisons. *Diagnostic and Statistical Manual of Mental Disorders.* 4th edition: 1999.

"Antidepressant potential of oral S-adenosyl-l-methionine." *Acta Psychiatrica.* 81, number 5 (1990 May): 432–436.

Archer, J. "Relationship between estrogen, serotonin, and depression." *Menopause.* 6, number 1 (1999 Spring): 71–78.

Archives of General Psychiatry. 55 (1998): 771–778.

Balch, James F., M.D., and Phyllis A. Balch, C.N.C. *Prescription For Nutritional Healing.* Avery, 1990.

Baldewicz, T. et al. "Plasma pyridoxine deficiency is related to increased psychological distress in recently bereaved homosexual men." *Psychosomatic Medicine.* 60, number 3 (1999 May): 297–308.

Bell, I. et al. Brief communication. "Vitamin B1, B2, and B6 augmentation of tricyclic antidepressant treatment in geriatric depression with cognitive dysfunction." *Journal of the American College of Nutrition.* 11, number 2 (1992 April): 159–163.

Benton, D. et al. "The effects of nutrients on mood." *Public Health Nutrition.* 2, number 3A (1999 September): 403–409.

Breggin, Peter. *Toxic Psychiatry.* St. Martin's Press, 1994.

Cardello, H. et al. "Measurement of the relative sweetness of stevia extract, aspartame and cyclamate/saccharin blend as compared to sucrose at different concentrations." *Plant Foods for Human Nutrition.* 54, number 2 (1999): 119–130.

Caruso, I. et al. "Double-blind study of 5-hydroxy troptophan versus placebo in the treatment of primary fibromyalgia syndrome." *Journal of International Medical Research.* 18, number 3 (1990): 201–209.

Cecil, J. et al. "Relative contributions of intestinal, gastric, oro-sensory influences and information to changes in appetite induced by the same liquid meal." *Appetite.* 31, number 3 (1998 December): 377–390.

Chapman, I. et al. "Effects of small-intestinal fat and carbohydrate infusions on appetite and food intake in obese and non-obese men." *American Journal of Clinical Nutrition.* 69, number 1 (1999 January): 6–12.

"Clinical evaluation of S-adenosyl-L-methionine versus transcutaneous electrical nerve stimulation in primary fibromyalgia." *Current Therapeutic Research.* 53, number 2 (1993 February): 222.

"Clinical potential of ademetionine (S-adenosylmethionine) in neurological disorders." *Drugs.* 48, number 2 (1994): 137–152.

Connor, W. et al. "Increased docosahexaenoic acid levels in human newborn infants by administration of sardines and fish oil during pregnancy." *Lipids.* Supplemental. 31 (1996 March): S183–S187.

Damasio, A. "How the brain creates the mind." *Scientific American.* 281, number 6 (1999 December): 112–117.

"Depression and disability in Parkinson's disease." *Journal of Neuropsychiatry and Clinical Neurosciences.* 8 (1996): 20–25.

Di Benedetto, P. et al. "Clinical evaluation of SAMe versus transcutaneous nerve stimulation in primary fibromyalgia." *Current Therapeutic Research.* 53 (1993): 222–229.

"Double-blind, placebo-controlled study of S-adenosyl-L-methionine in depressed postmenopausal women." *Psychotherapy and Psychosomatics.* 59, number 1 (1993): 34–40.

Dowling, Colette. *You Mean I Don't Have To Feel This Way?* Charles Scribner's Sons, 1991.

Edwards, R. et al. "Omega-3 polyunsaturated fatty acid levels in the diet and in red blood cell membranes of depressed patients." *Journal of Affective Disorders.* 48, numbers 2–3 (1998 March): 149–155.

"Efficacy of S-adenosyl-L-methionine in speeding the onset of action of imipramine." *Psychiatry Research.* 44 (1992): 3.

"Evaluation of S-adenosylmethionine (SAMe) effectiveness on depression." *Current Therapeutic Research.* 27, number 6II (1980): 908–918.

"Evaluation of S-adenosylmethionine in primary fibromyalgia. A double-blind, crossover study." *American Journal of Medicine.* 83, number 5A (1987): 107–110.

"Evidence of depression provoked by cardiovascular medication: A prescription sequence symmetry analysis." *Epidemiology.* 7 (1996): 478–484.

Fugh-Berman, A. et al. "Dietary supplements and natural products as psychotherapeutic agents." *Psychosomatic Medicine.* 61, number 5 (1999 September–October): 712–728.

George, M. et al. "Transcranial magnetic stimulation: Applications in neuropsychiatry." *Archives of General Psychiatry.* 56, number 4 (1999 April): 300–311.

Gibson, R. et al. "Effect of dietary docosahexaenoic acid on brain composition and neural function in term infants." *Lipids.* Supplemental. 31 (1996 March): S177–S181.

Goleman, Daniel. "Costs of depression are on a par with heart disease, a study says." *The New York Times.* December 3, 1993.

Haleem, D. et al. "24-hour withdrawal following repeated administration of caffeine attenuates brain serotonin but not tryptophan in rat brain: Implications for caffeine-induced depression." *Life Sciences.* 57, number 19 (1995): PL285–PL292.

Hall, S. et al. "Nicotine, negative affect, and depression." *Journal of Consulting and Clinical Psychology.* 61, number 5 (1993 October): 761–767.

Hamazaki, T. et al. "The effect of docosahexaenoic acid on aggression in young adults: A placebo-controlled, double-blind study." *Journal of Clinical Investigation.* 97, number 4 (1996 February 15): 1129–1133.

Hawton, K. and L. Vislisel. "Suicide in nurses." *Suicide and Life Threatening Behavior.* 29, number 1 (1999 Spring): 86–95.

Healy, David. *The Antidepressant Era.* Harvard, 1998.

Heinz, A. et al. "Severity of depression in abstinent alcoholics is associated with monoamine metabolites and dehydroepiandrosterone-sulfate concentrations." *Psychiatry Research.* 89, number 2 (1999 December 20): 97–106.

Hoehn-Saric, R. et al. "Apathy and indifference in patients on fluvoxamine and fluoxetine." *Journal of Clinical Psychopharmacology.* 10, number 5 (1990): 343–345.

Horger, I. "Enzyme therapy in multiple rheumatic diseases." *Therapiewoche.* 33 (1983): 3948–3957.

Horrocks, L. and Y. Yeo. "Health benefits of docosahexaenoic acid (DHA)." *Pharmacology Research.* 40, number 3 (1999 September): 211–225.

Horvath, K. et al. "Gastrointestinal abnormalities in children with autistic disorder." *Journal of Pediatrics.* 135, number 5 (1999 November): 559–563.

Joffe, H. et al. "Estrogen, serotonin, and mood disturbance: Where is the therapeutic bridge?" *Biological Psychiatry.* 1(44), number 9 (1998 November): 798–811.

The Johns Hopkins Medical Institute. *The Johns Hopkins White Papers.* Baltimore, Maryland: 1999.

Jorgensen, M. et al. "Visual acuity and erythrocyte docosahexaenoic acid status in breast-fed and formula-fed term infants during the first four months of life." *Lipids.* 31, number 1 (1996 January): 99–105.

Journal of the American Academy of Child and Adolescent Psychiatry. 38 (1999): 1271–1276.

Journal of the American Medical Association. 277 (1997): 333.

Koob, G. and S. Heinrichs. "A role for corticotropin releasing factor and urocortin in behavioral responses to stressors." *Brain Research.* 848, numbers 1–2 (1999 November 27): 141–152.

Koroleva, V. et al. "Hippocampal damage induced by carbon monoxide poisoning and spreading depression is alleviated by chronic treatment with brain derived polypeptides." *Brain Research.* 816, number 2 (1999 January 23): 618–627.

Lam, R. et al. "A controlled study of light therapy in women with late luteal phase dysphoric disorder." *Psychiatry Research.* 86, number 3 (1999 June 30): 185–192.

Leary, Warren. "Depression travels in disguise with other illness." *The New York Times.* January 17, 1996.

Ledochowski, M. et al. "Fructose malabsorption is associated with early signs of mental depression." *European Journal of Medical Research.* 3, number 6 (1998 June 17): 295–298.

Lydiard, R. and S. Falsetti. "Experience with anxiety and depression treatment studies: Implications for designing irritable bowel syndrome clinical trials." *American Journal of Medicine.* 107, number 5A (1999 November 8): 65S–73S.

Lipton, M. et al. "Vitamins, megavitamin therapy and the nervous system." *Nutrition and the Brain.* Volume 3. Raven Press. (1979): 183–264.

Linde, K. et al. "St. John's wort for depression: An overview and meta-analysis of randomized clinical trials." *British Medical Journal.* (1996 August 3).

Lucas, A. et al. "Breast-milk and subsequent intelligence quotient in children born pre-term." *Lancet.* 339 (1992): 261–264.

McLeod, M. et al. "Chromium potentiation of antidepressant pharmacotherapy for dysthymic disorder in 5 patients." *Journal of Clinical Psychiatry.* 60, number 4 (1999 April): 237–240.

Makrides, M. et al. "Effect of maternal docosahexaenoic acid (DHA) supplementation on breast milk composition." *European Journal of Clinical Nutrition.* 50, number 60 (1996 June): 352–357.

Miller, G. et al. "Pathways linking major depression and immunity in ambulatory female patients." *Psychosomatic Medicine.* 61, number 6 (1999 November–December): 850–860.

"Monitoring S-adenosyl-methionine blood levels and antidepressant effect." *Acta Neurologica.* 35, number 6 (1980): 488–495.

Murray, Michael T. and Joseph E. Pizzorno. *An Encyclopedia of Natural Medicine.* Prima Publishing, 1991.

Murray, Michael T. *Natural Alternatives to Over-the-Counter and Prescription Drugs.* William Morrow and Company Incorporated, 1994.

Murray, Michael. *Natural Alternatives to Prozac.* William Morrow and Company, 1996.

"Neuroendocrine effects of S-adenosyl-(L)-methionine, a novel putative antidepressant." *Journal of Psychiatric Research.* 24 (1990): 2.

Nicolodi, M. and F. Sicuteri. "Fibromyalgia and migraine, two faces of the same mechanism. Serotonin as the common clue for pathogenesis and therapy." *Advanced Experimental Medicine and Biology.* (1996): 373–379.

NIH Depression Awareness, Recognition, and Treatment (D/ART) Program. American Psychiatric Association. Drug Facts and Comparisons. *Diagnostic and Statistical Manual of Mental Disorders.* 4th edition: 1999.

Nolen-Hoeksema et al. "Explaining the gender difference in depressive symptoms." *Journal of Personality Social Psychology.* 77, number 5 (1999 November): 1061–1072.

Norden, Michael J. *Beyond Prozac.* Regan Books, 1996.

"Oral S-adenosylmethionine in depression: A randomized, double-blind, placebo-controlled trial." *American Journal of Psychiatry.* 147, number 5 (1990 May): 591–595.

"Oral S-adenosyl-L-methionine in depression." *Current Therapeutic Research.* (1992 September): 478–485.

Pauling, Linus. *How to Live Longer and Feel Better.* W. H. Freeman and Company, 1986.

Peet, M. et al. "Depletion of omega-3 fatty acid levels in red blood cell membranes of depressive patients." *Biological Psychiatry.* 43, number 5 (1998 March 1): 315–319.

Richards, D. et al. "Stimulation of auricular acupuncture points in weight loss." *Australian Family Physician.* Supplemental 2. 27 (1998 July): S73–S77.

RochadeMelo, A. et al. "Spreading depression is facilitated in adult rats previously submitted to short episodes of malnutrition during the lactation period." *Brazilian Journal of Medical and Biological Research.* 30, number 5 (1997): 663–669.

Ross, Harvey M. *Fighting Depression.* Keats Publishing, 1992.

Ryman, Danielle. *Aromatherapy.* Bantam Books, 1993.

"S-adenosylmethionine blood levels in major depression: Changes with drug treatment." *Acta Neurologica Scandanavia Supplementum.* 89. number 154 (1994): 15–18.

"S-adenosyl-L-methionine in the treatment of major depression complicating chronic alcoholism." *Current Therapeutic Research, Clinical and Experimental.* 55 (1994): 1.

Salin-Pascual, R. and R. Drucker-Colin. "A novel effect of nicotine on mood and sleep in major depression." *Neuroreport.* 9, number 1 (1998 January 5): 57–60.

Sears, Barry. *The Zone.* Regan Books, 1995.

Semendeferi, K. et al. "The brain and its main anatomical subdivisions in living hominoids using magnetic resonance imaging." *Journal of Human Evolution.* 38, number 2 (2000 February): 317–332.

Schultz, H. and M. Jobert. "Effects of hypericum extract on the sleep EEG in older volunteers." *Journal of Geriatric Psychiatry and Neurology.* 7 (1994): S39–S43.

Sheppard, K. *Food Addiction.* 2nd ed. Heath Communication, 1993.

Shibata, H. et al. "Relationship of serum cholesterols and vitamin E to depressive status in the elderly." *Journal of Epidemiology.* 9, number 4 (1999 August): 261–267.

Shimizu, K. et al. "Suppression of glucose absorption by extracts from the leaves of *Gymnema inodorum.*" *Journal of Veterinary Medical Science.* 59, number 9 (1997 September): 753–757.

Slagle, Patricia. *The Way Up From Down.* Random Books, 1987.

Smith, Janie. "Sleep deprivation helps treat depression." *Let's Live.* (1988 September): 79.

Smyth, Angela. *Seasonal Affective Disorder.* Harper Collins Publishers, 1991.

Soderberg, M. et al. "Fatty acid composition of brain phospholipids in aging and in Alzheimer's disease." *Lipids.* 26 (1991): 421–425.

Sperber, A. et al. "Fibromyalgia in the irritable bowel syndrome: Studies of prevalence and clinical implications." *American Journal of Gastroenterology.* 94, number 12 (1999 December): 3541–3546.

Steinberg, S. et al. *Biological Psychiatry.* 45, number 3 (1999 February 1): 313–320.

Stevens, Laura J. et al. "Essential fatty acid metabolism in boys with attention-deficit, hyperactivity disorder." *American Journal of Clinical Nutrition.* 62 (1995): 761–768.

Tracy, Ann Blake. *Prozac Panacea or Pandora.* Cassia Publications, 1994.

"Treatment of depression in rheumatoid arthritic patients. A comparison of S-adenosylmethionineand placebo in a double-blind study." *Clinical. Trials Journal.* 24, number 4 (1987): 305–310.

Trikas, P. et al. "Core mental state in irritable bowel syndrome." *Psychosomatic Medicine.* 61, number 6 (1999 November–December): 781–788.

Van, R. et al. "Selenium deficiency in total parenteral nutrition." *American Journal of Clinical Nutrition.* 32 (1979): 2076–2085.

Vatn, M. "Food intolerance and psychosomatic experience." *Scandavian Journal of Work, Environment and Health.* Supplemental 3. 23 (1997): 75–78.

Wade, T. et al. "Anorexia nervosa and major depression: Shared genetic and environmental risk factors." *American Journal of Psychiatry.* 157, number 3 (2000 March): 469–471.

Walters, E. et al. "Bulimia nervosa and major depression: Common genetic and environmental factors." *Psychological Medicine.* 22, number 3 (1992 August): 617–622.

Weil, Andrew, M.D. *Natural Health, Natural Medicine.* Houghton Mifflin Company, 1990.

"When cholesterol does not satisfy." *American Journal of Clinical Nutrition.* 62 (1995): 1–9.

Williams, L. et al. "Quantitative association between altered plasma esterified omega-6 fatty acid proportions and psychological stress." *Prostaglandins Leukotrienes and Essential Fatty Acids.* 47, number 2 (1992 October): 165–170.

Worthington, J. et al. "Consumption of alcohol, nicotine, and caffeine among depressed outpatients. Relationship with response to treatment." *Psychosomatics.* 37, number 6 (1996 November–December): 518–522.

Wright, K. et al. "Caffeine and light effects on nighttime melatonin and temperature levels in sleep-deprived humans." *Brain Research.* 747, number 1 (1997 January 30): 78–84.

Wurtman, Richard J. and Judith J. "Brain serotonin, carbohydrate-craving, obesity and depression." *Advanced Experimental Medicine and Biology.* 398 (1996): 35–41.

Wurtman, Richard J. and Judith J. "Carbohydrates and depression." *Scientific American.* (1989 January): 68–75.

Wyatt, K. et al. "Efficacy of vitamin B-6 in the treatment of premenstrual syndrome: Systematic review." *BMJ: British Medical Association.* 318, number 7195 (1999 May 22): 1375–1381.

Yudofsky, Stuart, Robert Hales and Tom Ferguson. *What You Need to Know About Psychiatric Drugs.* Grove Widenfield, 1991.

Zucker, Martin. "Food and mood—There's no mistaking the connection." *Let's Live.* (1988 December): 12–22.

Index

About the Author

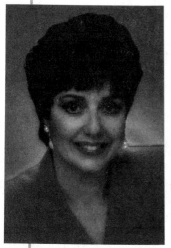

RITA ELKINS, M.H., has worked as an author and research specialist in the health field for the last ten years, and possesses a strong background in both conventional and alternative health therapies. She is the author of numerous books, including *The Complete Home Health Advisor,* which combines standard medical treatments with holistic alternatives for more than 100 diseases, *The Pocket Herbal Reference, The Complete Fiber Fact Book,* and *The Herbal Emergency Guide.* Rita has also authored dozens of booklets exploring the documented value of natural supplements like SAMe, noni, blue-green algae, chitosan, stevia and many more. She received an honorary Master Herbalist Degree from the College of Holistic Health and Healing in 1994.

Rita is frequently consulted for the formulation of herbal blends and has recently joined the 4-Life Research Medical Advisory Board. She is a regular contributor to *Let's Live* and *Great Life* magazines and is a frequent host on radio talk shows exploring natural health topics. She lectures nationwide on the science behind natural compounds and collaborates with medical doctors on various projects. Rita's publications and lectures have been used by companies like Nature's Sunshine, 4-Life Research, Enrich, NuSkin, and Nutraceutical to support the credibility of natural and integrative health therapies. She recently co-authored *Soy Smart Health* with *New York Times'* best-selling author Neil Solomon, M.D.

Rita resides in Utah, is married, and has two daughters and two granddaughters.

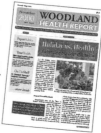